The Country Doctor's Wife is a surprisingly humorous, incredibly poignant first-person account of life in rural Ohio in the 1920s and 1930s. Cornelia Cattell Thompson, the wife of country doctor, Jay Ira Thompson, tells us in her own vibrant words about the challenges of living both in the shadows and at the center of her husband's vocation. In rich, well-crafted details, the well-educated Cornelia paints a vivid portrait of the daily life and death of the people who carved their existence out of this part of the eastern Ohio landscape. Angela Feenerty's judicious editing of this wonderful found manuscript allows Thompson's witty voice to come sparkling through page after page of this delightful book.

~Christina Fisanick, author of *Digital Storytelling as Public History*

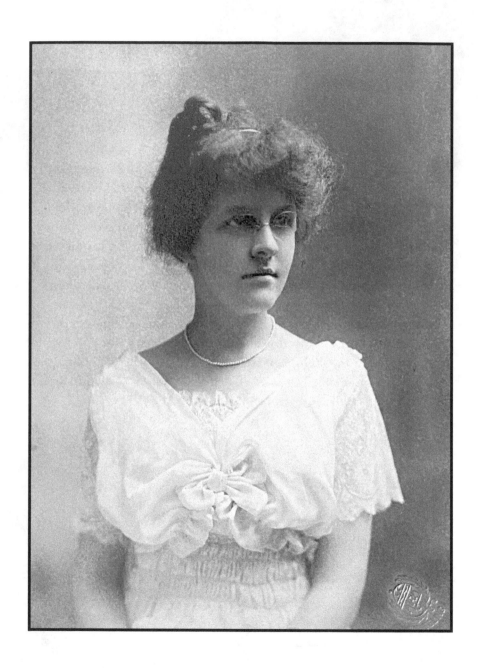

The Country Doctor's Wife

Memoir

Cornelia Cattell Thompson

Edited by Angela Feenerty

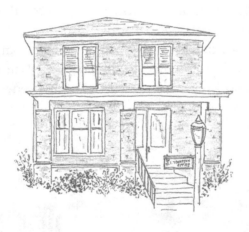

Appalachian Writing Series
Bottom Dog Press
Huron, OH 44839

Credits
Editor & Introduction: Angela Feenerty
General Editor & Introduction by Larry Smith
Cover art and design by Angela Feenerty

Acknowledgments
We thank the Historical Society of Mount Pleasant for the use of
photos and the Smithfield Historical Society for the image of the
doctor's sign.
Of course, we are indebted to Cornelia Cattell Thompson for keeping such detailed and human records of her place and time. The
press would also like to acknowledge Angela Feenerty's tireless efforts in transcribing and editing this book.

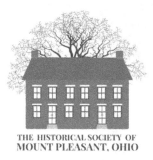

THE HISTORICAL SOCIETY OF
MOUNT PLEASANT, OHIO

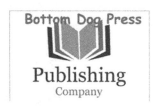

Publishing
Company

Contents

Introductions

I would have liked Cornelia Cattell Thompson. She was witty, ironic, and maybe a bit eccentric—my kind of person. When I visited Smithfield, just a few miles from historic Mount Pleasant, my feelings were cemented even more by the stories I heard from people who remembered her. Just snippets here and there—from Dave, who worked for Cornelia as a young man at the age 16, and now lives in the house she once called home, and Linda who met Cornelia and Nancy when Cornelia was considering selling her home. Cornelia escorted them to the second floor where she had just painted an array of lines and stripes on the bedroom floor and proclaimed it her masterpiece.

Her view on life was no doubt shaped by the early death of her mother to cancer, by the death of her beloved brother Ezra who died in the first world war—his body still lies in France where he died—by her Quaker upbringing, but also by her wide and open readings.

The Quakers, also known as Friends, came to Mount Pleasant early in the 19th century, and many remain today. From the chapter on Quakers she states that her grandmother was the last person in the church to wear the plain clothing associated with the 19th-century Quakers. (Ruthanna Cattell, her grandmother is seen in the family photograph in Quaker Plain dress.) But it was Cornelia's description of a Quaker funeral that most amused me.

Their church services have no elaborate ritual, nor have marriages or burials. I attended a Friend's funeral when I was ten. We sat and sat and silently contemplated the virtues of the dead (or our overpowering desire for roller skates). At last, the minister stood. He wore a benign countenance and a rusty frock coat. He folded his hands and preached the funeral sermon. I quote it complete:
"When James Eldridge sold a quart of beans—he sold a quart of beans."
The funeral was over.

I'm thankful that when Cornelia, and later Nancy, needed to find a home for her writings and their treasured memories, they chose to donate them to the Historical Society of Mount Pleasant, otherwise her unique story of a place and its people may have never been told.

~Angela Feenerty, president of the Historical Society of Mount Pleasant, Ohio

Imagine a woman of keen observation, a sharp ear, quick wit, and a great talent with words. Now place her in a tiny country town in Southern Ohio in the early 20th century, and mate her with a devoted husband serving as a country doctor. She not only keeps all home fires burning, but journeys with him in service to a lively community by patching up wounds, soaking up blood, assisting at baby births and neighbor deaths, and caring for families with her close listening. Like Ohio's other great homespun humorist, Erma Bombeck, Cornelia Cattell Thompson is a sharp-witted recorder of domestic life.

To our good fortune, Cornelia vividly records and shares those times, places, circumstances, and its many characters. Her ear for dialect and character comes with great humor as in this scene where she records her maid Susie's rant: "One husband is enough—too much salt spoils the soup—but we do need one. . . .When does a wife get her praise? In her casket with wife number two lookin' on. . . .The greatest trouble with men is that they develops a cessation of courtin'. They all say, 'I feeds you and I clothes you. What more do you want! Do I have to work all day and kiss you all night? I'm willin' to pay my fare after I ketch the streetcar, but I won't keep chasin' it.'"

Her style is clean and authentic yet alive to the humor and sorrow of everyday life, as well as its hidden beauty. She awakens us and makes life more precious because we sense how we could so easily miss it. She records one of many nights of being called out:

I took in at a glance—oil lamp, young child asleep on the iron bedstead, a blazing open fireplace surrounded with steaming clothes, three cats, two dogs, some tall cans of milk, a large basket of apples in the corner, bare floors, windows untrimmed except for frosted panes, wide borders of moonlight around the frames and drifts of white on the sills, and a woman in drab clothing huddled on a low stool near the fire. Jerry introduced me and said I had some experience as a nurse.

Here is a writing worthy of our attention, lyric with detail, wize from experience. Though most of it remained unpublished, and she clearly tried, it proves a most welcome gift to us all.

~Larry R. Smith, director of Bottom Dog Press

Engaged to a Country Doctor

[Cornelia Cattell Thompson (Feb. 5, 1898—May 31, 1982) was born in Wheeling, West Virginia. At age 2 her family moved to Martins Ferry, Ohio, and then in 1906 to Mount Pleasant, Ohio, where she attended school. Here her mother Edith died in 1913 when Cornelia was 14. A short time later, her father, William (1860—1931) moved his family from Mount Pleasant to nearby Smithfield, Ohio, where Cornelia would come to meet Dr. Jay Ira Thompson (Jan. 1891—Oct. 1955, an early graduate of The Medical School of Ohio State University 1914). Cornelia graduated at the head of her class from Mount Union College in Alliance, Ohio, in May of 1917. After graduation, she taught school, first in Carrollton, Ohio, and last in Barnesville, Ohio. She stopped teaching school shortly after her marriage in 1924 to Dr. Jay (Jerry) Thompson. She wrote all of her life, children's books, articles, and this running memoir of their life.]

The experience of being engaged to a Country Doctor with a busy established practice is not the same as that of a debutante who announces her engagement to someone of like station in the social register. Nor is it the same, I should think, as being engaged to an eager new physician so anxious for patients that each ring of a bell is a thrill. Jerry told me that when he made his first call on a seriously ill patient and told the family the patient was dying, he sat up all night watching for the undertaker scared silly that the patient would not die and yet oppressed with his inability to avert imminent death. After we met, we did not pray for patients, but that we might have an occasional evening when everyone would be well.

I had all sorts of warnings about the course the stars charted for us if we married. His invitations went something like this:

He, "Let's have dinner in Pittsburgh Thursday evening, go to the theater, and dance a bit—that is, if Mrs. M. accommodates us by having her baby before then."
(Mrs. M. selected Thursday to have her baby. No dinner, no theater, no dancing. Babies march on!)

He, "Would you mind going on alone to the dinner party? I have to make a call in G—. It's only 15 miles, so I'll not be very late."
(Attended dinner party alone. Came home alone. I began to see dim handwriting on the wall.)

He, "I think I can get away by nine for a movie tonight if you would like to go—that is—Oh! What's the use?"
(A movie? Don't make me laugh, and yet our movie-going stimulates the imagination as we seldom see both beginning and end.)

He, "I'll try to make it early for the bridge party tonight."
(They all smiled weakly as we arrived in time for two hands of bridge. Comforting thought—our house will never be furnished with bridge prizes.)

He, "I have tickets for Kreisler Friday night. You get the train at Wheeling and I'll catch it at East S."
(NO passenger entered at East S. No escort, no ticket, no Kreisler.)

I became well inured to arriving late for second courses at dinners, dances, movies, bridge parties, football games, but I never quite became accustomed to his being called out once we had arrived, as he usually was.

One morning Jerry was summoned from church to an accident. We left and en route home saw my father's car being hauled in by the wrecking car. We found him badly hurt. A drunken driver, in a new car with no insurance, had hit his car which was filled with young children he was driving to the Children's Home from Sunday School.

Sometimes I sat alone through movies, or whatever it was—often he returned. While I was still teaching, I would dash into a neighboring city to meet him for dinner and the theater. I could describe every hotel lobby in a radius of fifty miles down to the last palm and fat Buddha lamp. By the time he arrived, we usually had to miss either dinner or the show, so the choice depended on when we'd last eaten. We had dinner and arrived early for "A Blossom Time," but he slept through it, having had no sleep in forty hours.

When I became ill in the town where I was teaching, he arrived unannounced at 3 A.M., bundled me up and took me home. I thought how wonderful it was going to be to have a doctor for a husband. I now buy my aspirin at the garage up the street or pilfer samples from the morning mail. He hears complaints all day and much of the night, and garage aspirin is effective enough.

One evening we were dancing at a local party. Jerry was called to the door and returned saying, "I believe I'll have to go—woman sick. Don't think I'll be long, so why not go along?"

It was a beautiful night and heavy chains helped us to plow through the deep snow. The house was in the country about eight miles distant. I wore boots and a heavy fur coat and had a blanket to keep me warm while I waited in the car. He was gone so long that I fell asleep. When he woke me it was much later. "Awfully sorry, but I'm in more, or less of a jam and can't leave to take you home. The patient is having a baby. There is no one in there to help except her husband. I hate to ask you, but do you suppose you could help me for a while?"

I assured him overconfidently that I was practically an obstetrician in a previous incarnation, and then waded through snow up to my quivering knees. My erstwhile pose as a brittle young modern, armed to the teeth with information about the Why's and Wherefore's of Life and its processes dissolved like Jell-O in hot water. I hoped silently that I'd slip and break a leg, or at least sprain an ankle, which is one of my accomplishments at less opportune times. I took a hasty last look at the lovely moon, so clean, so white, so pure, so innocent, so far removed from cataclysms on the Planet Earth.

We stamped off what snow we could on the small porch and had no difficulty entering the front door. It would not close but gaped wide open and the narrow beam of the flashlight showed a long sweep of snow in the dark hall. Jerry told me to keep on my coat and boots as we entered the room on the right.

I took in at a glance—oil lamp, young child asleep on the iron bed-stead, a blazing open fireplace surrounded with steaming clothes, three cats, two dogs, some tall cans of milk, a large basket of apples in the corner, bare floors, windows untrimmed except for frosted panes, wide borders of moonlight around the frames and drifts of white on the sills, and a woman in drab clothing huddled on a low stool near the fire. Jerry introduced me and said I had some experience as a nurse. All I could remember on the spur of the moment was my brothers' small ills—whooping cough, mumps, measles, broken arms, and the time at college when I found a postcard in the morning mail, on one side of which was the picture of a hospital on the other the words: "Dear Sis, I hope I don't die tomorrow. Charles." And the ensuing dash by taxi and train to make sure he wouldn't if I could help it. All our youthful small ills kaleidoscoped in my fevered brain as I faced this emergency.

The patient sat impassively by the fire with no flicker of interest in the proceedings, or in us. I soon discovered that Jerry had been trying to persuade her to go to bed, but she refused without sound—just sat. It was completely baffling. She wouldn't talk. Jerry said, "If you will please tell me when you are having pains, I can time them." No reply. It was weird. I sensed that he did not think the soiled calico dress and the long black cotton stockings the ideal outfit for the accouchement. He sent a despairing SOS in my direction. My training in music, experience in schoolroom management, and knowledge of foreign languages failed me in this emergency. Jerry and the soon-to-be papa went out to see about the water supply in the kitchen. I suddenly decided to try a practical application of Dramatics and Psychology.

"Men don't know how we (!) feel at a time like this, do they?"
"En how." (Expressionless)
"Would you mind if I would make a bed for your little girl on the
bench near the fire?"
"Nope."
I kept on chatting while I folded a thick black lumpy comfort on the
bench, flattened the lumps, lifted the little girl to her new bed.
"What a sweet little girl. I'm sure your new baby will be lovely, too."
"Fat chance."
My ardor was slightly dampened by this ambiguous remark, but I
smiled brightly as I made up her bed.
"Don't you think you would be more comfortable if you would lie
down?"
"Nope."
"Would you like me to help you undress?" (I supposed they undressed
to have a baby.)
"Nope."
When Jerry returned and found her lying on the bed—I don't yet
know how I did it he sighed aloud, then whispered to me.
"You should have a Carnegie medal."

I began the first of many treks to the distant kitchen, each one an
adventure in hardihood. I buttoned up my coat and hurried through
the snow-filled hall. My only light was an occasional lost moonbeam
and the flashlight hastily thrust in my hand. I could find no kitchen.
Opening the rear door, I saw a slim pencil of light around a door
about thirty feet distant. To reach it I crossed a snowy porch. The
wind nearly blew the old door off the rusty hinges when I opened it.
I found a battered coal stove burning lustily, seemingly aware of its
own important role. The room contained bare essentials: the stove, a
table, four chairs, a mongrel cupboard, and the fire-man papa sitting
in a tilted chair with feet propped on the oven door—a coal bucket
on each side of him. He used these alternately as a temporary resting
place for what seemed to be a constant stream of tobacco juice. He
made no offer to rise, but did play host saying, "Have a seat, Lady."
And I thought my arrival stimulated the number of spurts toward the
battered receptacles beside him. I wondered why the saturated coal

did not quench the fire. He was reveling in the safe distance between him and the scene of conflict. In contrast to the patient he chatted volubly.

"I guess this is the best place for me, Mrs. Dr. The last time she threw her shoes at me. You don't think he needs me in there do you, Lady? (hopefully) I'll keep the fire going and open doors for you. I don't mind missing a little sleep, do you, Lady?" (I didn't—then.)

"Does your wife have a nightgown?" I asked.

His ears got red, he looked at the floor, he scuffed his shoes on the oven grating.

"She used to have one of those things. It might be upstairs."

I urged him to find it and heard him tramping around overhead. He brought back an ancient flannelette nightgown with dark streaks on all the folds. I knew we could not wash it, but I brushed off a cobweb, shook it well, asked him to remove his feet from the oven temporarily, rolled it in a paper and laid it in the recently vacated oven to warm. After an exploratory trip to the bedroom-nursery-kennel, I returned the next time with the surprise wrapped in the newspaper. I handed it to Jerry with one quiet word, "Eureka." His appreciation of me mounted. This time he did not ask if she wished to don the garment. He simply undressed her as if she were a recalcitrant child, which she was, and asked me to pull the gown over her head when he lifted her, then he rolled off the long black stockings.

About 2 A.M. he called me aside, "I need some extra supplies. Would you rather take the man for company and drive to the office for them, or stay here while I go?" With no hesitation, I chose the former. The prospect of welcoming a new child while the Doctor might possibly be reclining in a snowdrift, roused chills of apprehension.

We skidded into town and hurried back safely with needed supplies, I, for one, hoping the need for them was history. A flapping chain kept saying—"I hope it's over, I hope it's over." I did not take the time to go out to tell my father where I was. I had a feeling he would think I should be home. When we returned, I asked the patient if she had some clothes for the baby. "Upstairs in dresser."

I took the flashlight and reconnoitered in the bitterly cold dark room upstairs. Finally, I found a package in the brown wrapping paper of a mail-order house. It had never been unwrapped, but I took it and an old blanket that looked clean back to the warm room. I unwrapped the package and found a few pieces of baby clothing. They were so cold that my hands became numb, or at least I thought that was the reason. I stretched a string from a chair to the mantle corner and hung up (some of the articles). I removed a steaming, smelly jacket from another string and spread out the old blanket. Jerry inquired for oil of any sort, but they had none, so he told me to put a dish of lard or tallow on the hearth. I do not like cats anyway, but when they began snooping around the dish of tallow... I picked them all up and none too gently set them in the snowy hall with a gesture reminiscent of the positive one Father used when he re-set us in church if we talked too much, or turned to study the fascinating labyrinth of white whiskers on the chin of the one who occupied the pew just behind. To me, those whiskers were Henry Wadsworth Longfellow on our first set of Authors, and I never felt that Father was justified in trying to preserve the appearances of piety during over-long services when so much of interest lay to the rear.

Several times during the night Jerry asked me if I wanted to go out for air, but I assured him that my frequent trips to the loose-leaf kitchen supplied all needed air. He expected me to faint, but there was not time. Three times I cleaned up the bed after the patient vomited. There were no clean sheets or covers. I resorted to newspapers and old cloths. The baby refused to cry or breathe. Jerry spanked it resoundingly and tried other measures: and when they did not bring the desired results, he placed a piece of sterile gauze over the small mouth and applied suction with his own. It was a satisfactory substitute for an aspirator. I was glad I didn't have to do it. The baby cried. He dropped some medicine in the eyes and then handed the naked body to me in a towel, "Take it over to the fire and oil it. I'm too busy to help you." With trembling fingers, I began the unaccustomed task. A new sound startled me, and I turned to see the little girl sitting bolt upright taking in the whole situation. I heard an explosion directed at the papa, "Take that child to the kitchen and leave it there." The child left the room screaming. I heard tramping on the porch. The new arrival's grandmother came in with a blast of cold air. She immediately took charge of my sketchily oiled newcomer. A large feather pillow was warmed at the fire, the baby was laid on this diagonally. The bottom of the pillow was turned up. Two corners were folded. Strips were torn from an old piece of muslin and the cocoon was wrapped securely from shoulders to feet with lap after lap of the torn strips. I learned that this was to start the baby growing straight after having been in a cramped position for some time. I did not inquire about the sanitary arrangements.

Not until weeks later did I know that the terrible hemorrhages which the patient had were not normal. That night is etched on my mind more clearly than any similar occasion since. I made all sorts of mental observations as I tried to follow unfamiliar directions during the infinitely long night. I wondered if the fond father would throw out his chest the next day and hand out chewin' tobaccy to the neighbors. His role of firing the stove, eating apples, and chewing tobacco that he whittled from a sinister-looking bar about a foot long, (he advised me where to buy it to save money) seemed a very minor one to me. I now know that this observation was incorrect. Having had a baby, I should prefer to be the one receiving all the attention and feeling like the center of the universe of confusion, rather than the harassed father, who is not of sufficient importance to be present when his child is born. For a short time, it permits one the orgy of a beautiful martyr complex normally inadvisable. When we were ready to leave, Jerry took a few notes for the birth certificate. Turning to the mother he inquired, "I don't suppose you have a name for your new daughter?" over the child's arms and tummy. "What was that queer name you called her?" (Pointing to me.)
"Cornelia."
"That'll be it—Cornelia Aurelia."
I thought Lobelia would be nice too, but I gulped and smiled, and we said goodnight. We astonished my family, who never verbally admitted the existence of the process of birth, by walking into breakfast.

My sweet family adapted themselves as best they could to the new horizon that blazed across their Quaker sky, ignited by daughter's fiancée. When Jerry told Father that he hoped I would marry him, Father, with firm eye and firmer kindness, said, "I like you very much. To be quite frank, I think you smoke too much and don't go to church enough, but I have great respect and regard for you with these exceptions, which I shall not mention again." And he never did.

Their love and confidence, bolstered with Quaker stoicism, had weathered the all-night vigil when we started out one evening to make a call en route to a dinner in an adjacent city.

Jerry was delayed in the house as usual. It was such a lovely night, bright with moonlight, that I got out of the car and wandered along the lane made picturesque by the shadows of the old rail fence. My reverie was interrupted by a window hastily raised and by Jerry's urgent voice, "Come quickly!"

I found an air of intense excitement in the house. He handed me a huge carving knife abruptly, "Take this and keep it for me. Stand over at the other side of the bed." He turned to the man whose eyes were blazing with anger. "And you get the hell out of here and stay out."

The man slunk out. On the bed lay a terrified little girl who looked to be about twelve years old. When Jerry turned back the covers, I saw a strange little object, unlike the other new baby I had recently seen. This one was so tiny that it lay in the palm of Jerry's hand when he picked it up. It was withered and brown and looked like an old piece of leather. Fortunately, it lived but a few minutes. Busy with the care of the little girl, he asked me to wrap the dead baby in something and remove it from the bed. The girl's mother came in weeping. We stayed all night because the child was seriously ill as well as terrorized. When toward dawn we were ready to go, a neighbor promised to stay to see that the father did not enter the room. There are times even yet when I wish I could forget the stark terror on the face of that little girl. On the way home I heard the rest of the story.

At the supper table, she complained of a stomachache. Her mother told her to go into the other room and lie down. When the mother went in after a short while, she discovered the child in labor. Completely surprised and thoroughly frightened she called a son and told him to go quickly for the doctor without telling his father. The baby was born a few minutes after Jerry arrived. When the father heard the first cry, he grabbed the large carving knife and rushed into the room shouting, "You goddam little bitch, I'll kill you."

Jerry knocked him against the wall with such force that the knife fell to the floor. The child told Jerry that she had slept with an uncle for years. I have never seen him more affected by any case than he was by this one. For a time as we drove home, neither of us could speak. We had completely forgotten the party. At length, he broke the silence.

"That was a pretty stiff jolt for you. I don't mind telling you it knocked me out. I'll protect you all I can from the seamy side of this business, but it's rocky at best. You still have a week to change your mind and I wouldn't blame you."

We were married a week later. Having left town so that Jerry could be sure of being present at his own wedding.

We Acquire Possessions

After I finished teaching and came home, I found the days extremely busy ones. We could find no suitable house. There was one which appealed to me because of its long windows with very wide sills just off the floor, but Jerry insisted that we would be seasick from the uneven floors and that the log cabin part of the house was more quaint than practical.

Not over six houses in the town had modern conveniences and these would not have been given over without a death struggle, so we decided to build. Jerry laughingly said that he had to build a house to match my lovely linens and the fine quilts which I had made. These were being quilted by three of the local churches at *one cent* a yard, which seemed to me a slow way to further the work of the Lord, conscious as I was of pricked fingers and weary backs.

We had almost no money. There was no FHA. Neither of us knew anything about building houses, nor did we know what we wanted. My mental picture of what we needed was tall white columns outside and a bathroom inside. We look back in amazement at our early trepidations. As I recall the circumstances, our one hazy idea was to build as much house for as little money as possible. It never occurred to us to hire an architect. I made a rough sketch of what we thought we wanted, and the estimate was $22,000. Our wants changed instantly. Tall white columns metamorphosed into plain brick pillars; rooms vanished.

We called in a carpenter who was a skilled workman and who—blessed thought—owed Jerry a tremendous bill for medical services over a period of several years. He finally drew up the plans and the house was started.

Jerry was seldom around when a decision was to be made concerning the building. The carpenter-architect would consult me with no intention of listening. In deference to his deafness, I would shout a suggestion about height of cupboards, lift of stairs et cetera and he would fix me with the eye of a Cyclops, expel a large quantity of tobacco juice generally northeast of where I was standing (with occasional unpleasant detours), and shout, "Jesus Rivers! How many houses have *you* built? Well, I've built three hundred. I ought to know by this time that twelve inches is deep enough for cupboard shelves." The fact that I was to be solo housekeeper and at least co-owner of the house, mattered not at all when his judgment was in question. When Jerry would come and repeat my request firmly as if it had sprung like Venus from his masculine brain, the idea was carried out like magic.

There was one day when I doubted that I would ever occupy the house. I went with the carpenter and his daughter to town to select some fittings. His car was an old right-hand drive model—I'm sure I should feel uneasy in England. He drove in the middle of the road with no respect for traffic, curves, or warnings. If there had been green and red lights, he would have ignored them from principle and quoted the Constitution—Incorrectly. As we approached a narrow culvert, we distinctly heard the whistle of an approaching street car. The car track and the road through the culvert were synonymous. His daughter yelled. I yelled. We begged him to stop. When he finally heard a commotion from the rear, he jammed on all the brakes he had, I judged there were about fifty from my position on the floor. He turned a baleful eye and bellowed, "Jesus Rivers! Who's drivin' this car, you'r me. Now keep shut up and don't hinder progress."

His remarks were cut short by the screams of the brakes on the streetcar. They must have been good for we felt only a slight bump. After reversing ungracefully and letting the streetcar go on its merry way, we were speechless for a time. We crossed two sets of tracks without a passing glance in either direction or any slacking in the speed. There was one car ahead of us which seemed to annoy our driver. Finally, he wearied of the chase, speeded his motor and pulled out to turn. From his sheltered position on the right, he could not observe the long procession of cars approaching us—quite visible to me, I shouted but he pulled directly into the path of a hearse—significant I thought. The funeral procession was stopped while we got out to see if there were any damage to cars or corpse.

By this time I wondered if I really wanted a new house. Neither car was much damaged so on we sped to the city, they to the cemetery. We paid no heed to stop or cross streets. In the center of the business district he started blithely down a one-way street. Pedestrians scuttled and shrieked. The shattered occupants of the rear seat shouted. When an irate officer stepped on the running board, we stopped so abruptly that he lost his balance. He had previously lost his patience.

Someway we lived through that day. I longed to refuse transportation home but thought perhaps if I sat shivering and prayed…
En route home there was a very long, steep hill with a sharp turn at the very bottom. Just before the sharp turn were main line railroad tracks. In order to get a run for the hill, our driver stepped on the gas. I heard a train whistle. I'm not good at estimating distances, but thought we would be hit. The driver did not become alarmed because he neither heard nor saw. The train was backing up which probably saved our lives. I saw two men on the caboose platform cover their faces with their hands. The word Predistination flashed in my mind. I wished I were a Presbyterian. We made it—by inches.

There were no other tracks to cross or I should have walked, hoping for cooperation from uncertain knees. We were very silent for the remainder of the journey. That evening I begged to be excused from deciding the color of tile for the roof. The decision did not seem paramount.

I still chuckle about the time after the completion of the house, when good friend carpenter showed the house to some friends of his own and smiled as they admired the special features which he had convinced himself were the products of his own ingenuity.

He was an excellent workman—the house is still in fine condition—but if he could have had his way unhampered, it would be an 1890 sentinel to his memory.

I had inherited some fine family furniture and so decided to lean toward the colonial trend in decoration. The craze had not hit this section of the country, fortunately for me, so I was able to buy nearly anything I needed. After finding numerous things in the little Quaker town where I spent my girlhood, I persuaded Jerry to go with me to collect them. I longed even then for a camera record of that trip, in color. Today it would be priceless. I don't remember why we didn't hire a truck to go for the things, carrying me as chief guide. Many times since, I have ridden in various lumbering trucks to gather up stones for paths, topsoil, furniture, locust posts, but never with Jerry as chauffeur.

Once I drove a borrowed truck and took along an elderly woodsman who knew where to find material for rustic arbors. We started down a long, narrow hill, and I saw him put his hand over his eyes and push his muddy boots against the floor boards. "Are you afraid of my driving?" I modestly inquired.
Without removing his hand from his eyes, he weakly replied, "Well, not ezactly, Mrs., but I'm what you might call a leaner." I know just how he felt.

The only truck Jerry could commandeer for the furniture-gathering expedition was the delivery truck owned by a good friend who had the village meat market. It was small and geared to slow travel, a Model T Ford, of the vintage that required one to hold down a foot pedal, if he aspired to mount to the summit of a hill. The nine miles to the village of our destination is all hills. We never got the speed up to fifteen miles an hour. It averaged eight. Jerry seldom drives under fifty. After the first few miles he tried to be gay but I imagined his eyes were bloodshot. He began to question me about the treasures we were to gather up but I brightly changed the subject by calling attention to the dogwood in rampant bloom. Even then, I knew his powers of visualization were limited.

At the first stop, we collected from our old barn a seatless ladder back chair with one slat missing and two large copper kettles completely black from oxidation and disuse. Jerry had an expression on his face unfamiliar to me then. I have seen it since, when he collects me and new treasures at auctions. The next stop produced a spinning wheel (50c), a rosewood settee, ($2.00 without the seat), and two small Windsor rockers covered with red house paint (50c each). I thought Jerry was going to ask for his diamond back but he steadied himself by lighting a cigarette. I wonder if I started the chain habit!

We next picked up a candle stand, the top of which had rotted through from the moisture of thrifty geraniums in the village bank windows. This had been my grandmother's and to me was a great treasure. I thought it best not to ask Jerry's opinion. On to a damp basemen—we picked up a spool bed covered with green and blue mold in lovely shades ($3.00) and a day bed (free) in the same design and condition. Also an old Terry clock ($1.00) which contained in its yellowed interior a record of dates on which new calves might be expected.

We started home and Jerry rattled up to a small restaurant. I asked for ice cream and he said briefly, "Four cups of black coffee." The trip home was not particularly lively. I even began to question my own judgment. My only encouragement was that I knew we had eight rooms to furnish and no money for new furniture. To amuse myself, I tried to single out the pork odor from the beef, while he pumped the foot pedal and the copper kettles clanged like an ambulance. As he unloaded me and the booty, he said expressively, "I hope you are right. I GUESS I love you in spite of it."

Some of the villagers were not so kind. At local sales they smiled at each other when I would buy an old cherry two-drawer stand for 25c. The auctioneer relied on me, because he too thought that I would buy what no one else wanted. Once in a crowded house when he couldn't see me, he shouted: "Cornelia must be here. Cornelia, where

are you? Here's a pair of pewter candlesticks for you." When I offered
a dime, he said, "Sold," and they were handed back to me via fifty
odd hands. They proved to be holders for gas mantels. The town has
never had gas.

One well-intentioned lady of the village came to call. I learned the
real purpose of her call when she said: "Dearie, I feel I must advise
you since you have no mother. The whole town thinks it is a shame
for you to be fixing up all that old junk when the Doctor is building
you such a fine home."
I poured more tea as I tried to combine hospitality with tact and daz-
zling charm, but steered clear of a commitment.

Another evangel looked at my beautiful walnut cupboard and said,
"Too bad it has that crack."
I studied her numerous ones.
"Oh, but I can't agree with you there at all. This cupboard has per-
sonality. After all, most of us have cracks in our veneer somewhere,
if we've lived."

After a first scandalized look, she quickly recovered and made a
soothing remark. I felt as if she had dropped a peanut in my trunk
but knew she was either sympathizing with Jerry or questioning his
judgment.

An entire storeroom back of Father's house was given over to my
efforts at refinishing furniture. There were chairs and chests, beds,
tables and mirror frames. They had lived long but had not kept up. I
reeked of varnish remover and stain.

Jerry was constantly heard to remark, "Tomorrow I'll try to help you."
In my exuberant innocence I thought he meant it. One evening I persuaded him to try to sand down a table. He had just seized the sand-
ing block with an Indian club grip and made several deep scratches
in the smooth surface when he was called away. There was a gleam in
his eye as he hurried away faster than I thought necessary. Since that
time, I have learned that there is a very special fate in charge of the

destiny of M.D.'s. There is always someone desperately in need of help whenever M.D. in question is about to undertake something that does not lie within the orbit of his talents or inclinations.

The furniture began to look very well, and Jerry's spirits lightened. He was delighted that we were not going to be forced to camp in an empty house for an indefinite period. I made pillows out of a feather mattress, lamps out of old jugs and vases. It was fun. I had bought a barrel of dishes through friends who owned a pottery, but when I saw an Indian Tree design which I liked much better, I persuaded a store to trade, even though I had not bought the first ones there. My loyalty to that store never wavered.

We gave each other practical gifts on all occasions. I even gave Jerry a dozen Sterling butter knives for his birthday! When he wrote me from Boston where he was doing some post-graduate work at Harvard, that he had found a perfect watch set with diamonds, I answered that I thought we could eat better with knives and forks in our pattern, than with diamonds.

Aunt Lydia thought I should fill a handsome cedar chest, acquired with honest intentions during a previous love affair, with gifts similarly acquired and return it to the giver, but I procrastinated and it has been so useful for blankets!

Father gave us the piano. I was nine when the family acquired it and moved the square rosewood one to the third floor. I remember when Mother asked me, "Would you rather have a new piano, or a new baby sister?" And I immediately answered, "A piano." We got it—and a baby brother.

I had my eye on twin tables with lovely carved legs, but we bought a small gateleg table to use until we could afford the others. A very good friend bought them before we made the grade! I tried to get the rosewood organ which mother had loaned to a dear friend, who later died. Her husband offered to sell it to me for forty dollars.

One can learn a lot about human nature in the pursuit of old furniture. We had a fine old cherry bed and I went back to our old home to get its twin which we had left in the barn rafters. The new owner of the property said, "Oh, I sold that to the junk man for a dollar."

An elderly lady who had no other source of income agreed to knit rugs for one bedroom. She also sold me a hand knit room size rug, which she had made for herself, for twelve dollars. It was perfect for the dining room. I worry now that she has lost her sight. A patient made four braided rugs for the guest room, out of materials which I had dyed in several blending shades of rose. They were the right background for the guest room furniture, for which I had spent a total of $5.60.

Dressing table (no extra charge for red barn paint)	.25
Walnut stool	.10
Poster spool bed (moldy walnut)	3.00
Windsor rocker	.25
Ladder-back straight chair, which had been a rocker	0
Chest	2.00

I spent one day gathering up Jerry's possessions at his previous quarters and was mildly stunned to find 179 socks and 88 ties. I mentally figured how much cement and bricks that would have bought. Jerry said, "I always like to have enough of everything." With regard to sox and ties he had succeeded, but I understand because that is exactly how I felt about furnishing the house.

We spent approximately $1,000 for new possessions, chief of which were a down-filled davenport and unmatching Cogswell chair, good springs and mattresses, a modest gate leg table and Windsor chairs for the dining room.

I would do all of it again, although refinishing spool beds requires the patience of Job and recalls the copy book maxim, "If at first you don't succeed, try, try again." I shall never forget Jerry's immense surprise and pleasure that the 'old things' looked so well. He forgot his skepticism and we reveled in our beautiful home.

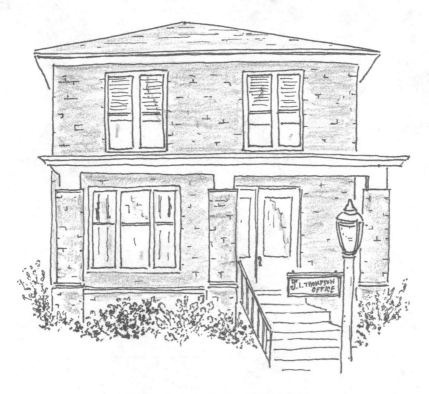

67 Maple Avenue, Smithfield, Ohio
*Art by Allen Frost

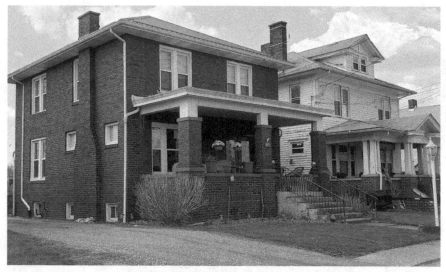

Houses in 2021, home at 67 Maple Ave. Smithfield and second house (right) that later served as doctor's office and Cornelia's antique shop.

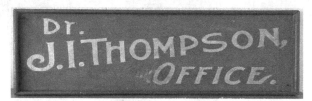

Original Office Sign

Mrs. Jerry Thompson

Antiques

Smithfield, Ohio 43948

Phone:
733-7020

Cornelia Cattelle Thompson

Through the Doctor's Eyes

[With the expansion of the railroad and the opening of coal mines came waves of immigrants. The July 9, 1891, Steubenville *Gazette* reported, "Mt. Pleasant people have come to realize that railroad civilization is very different from the classically cultured civilization that was obtained in this township in the old days." This cultural bias towards immigrants is apparent in some of Cornelia's writing. Hungarian, Italian and Czech miners poured into Eastern Ohio. As a rule, they didn't get along with one another, and didn't like the African American population who also gravitated towards the coal mines. Many of the African Americans living in the southwestern corner of Jefferson County, where Mount Pleasant and Smithfield are located, descended from former slaves of Ann Talliferro, who freed her slaves in 1854, and of Thomas Benford, who had freed his slaves in the 1830s. Charlotte Pollard, mentioned below was an emancipated slave of Ann Talliferro.]

Up to the time of our marriage I had been in Smithfield only brief periods between college [Mount Union] and teaching. Father had accepted a business offer, and moved here because both he and I felt that the small town would be the ideal place for my younger brothers—heaven forgive us. The rural school system nearly wrecked the mild beginnings of their education. Its inadequacy shocked me, but the years have brought improvements. Father's sister Lydia, blessed with compassion and infinite patience, kept the home fires intact while I was away. The house was not always dusted, but the baseball covers were mended and so, the boys were happy.

In my brief contacts, the town had impressed me superficially as a rather sleepy little place with uninteresting architecture and no evidence of interest in gardening as an art—the type of small town one passes through hurriedly when touring and then wonders if he has passed it. I had not then developed the unfortunate but inevitable X-ray eyes through which the doctor and his family see people and unfolding events.

I suppose we are the proverbial American cross-section, but for such a small place we do have many contrasting elements.

Our town's greatest tragedy is the wanton destruction by the so-called strip mines. Acre after acre has been gutted, the land permanently ruined. The dirt is stripped off so that the coal can be scooped up with shovels. Everything in the path of the coal vein is destroyed. Great oak woods have been felled. I cannot express what a shock it is to return to a favorite woods and find it gone, as we have done several times. Farms are ruined. Farmhouse after farmhouse stands vacant because the land is no longer tillable. The land is valueless when they have removed the coal and left mile after mile of serpentine gaping wounds. The latest news is that one of the companies is bringing in a shovel that will move over 300 bushels at one gulp. (It is here.) I have not seen lands desolated by modern warfare, but it would require a tremendous number of bombs to wreak the desolation of just one of the "sunshine mines." I shudder to think that the Divine Plan which so obviously produced Ohio with its lovely hills, valleys, woods, and streams, can be so ruthlessly defiled.

We are in the bituminous coal belt, so miners and their families make up a large group. Part of this group is definitely a community asset. Some own their homes and try thriftily to prepare for the inevitable strikes and business depressions. The ones who combat these difficulties most successfully are those who own small or large pieces of land on which they keep a few pigs, a cow, and some chickens and have space to raise most of their food. In this way, when the mines are working, they can save against a rainy day. I admire their thrift and industry.

One family is an interesting case in point. The father and mother acquired an old farm and as the son and daughters have married, they have built small homes on the same land. All are neat and well planted. Both the men and the women are industrious. The latter work in the mines whenever possible, but keep the gardens, stock and orchards cared for at all times. Theirs is the happy solution to the problem of social unrest resulting from labor troubles.

Many of the working class have drifted into the mines because of propinquity and a lack of preparation for skilled work of any sort. For many years it was an unusual occurrence for any young person to go to college.

Then we have a large group of miners, who have settled here like poisonous mushrooms, coming a circuitous route from less profitable coal fields. They are often shiftless and improvident. They present serious problems. Their children are taken into our schools. Health problems are acute. Rickets, skin diseases, tuberculosis, and social diseases are common. Many are a public charge for food and clothing. During strikes, they pad the relief rolls. At times they have become very troublesome because they feel they are not receiving their just dues. This attitude is reflected in that of a young man who decided to leave his work with us to go to the mines. I said, "But there will soon be a strike and at the best, work is uncertain." His reply: "That won't matter. That's why I'm leaving. They'll feed us. They have to."

I recall one young woman, aged 28, who grew tired of her legal mate and assumed another. She became pregnant. When her pains started, she walked to the home of her mother-in-law to which haven her husband had previously retired. For some time, she sat and talked as if it were an ordinary call, but gradually it was impressed upon the spectators that the birth of a child was imminent. They summoned the doctor. He was preceded by the arrival of husband and of adopted husband. Both staged a sit-down strike. The baby arrived. Jerry asked who the father of the child was. Number Two said, "I am." Number one volunteered, "Don't mind me, Doc, I'm only the husband."

In contrast, we have a group of colored families who have been assimilated into the village and community life. They are descendants of the intrepid slaves who escaped into Ohio via the underground railway, aided by my grandfather and other conscientious Quakers, who gave concrete evidence of their belief in freedom of the individual. They are, as a rule, honest, industrious, and thoroughly dependable.

In this group are many whose ancestors were freed by two southern gentlemen who sent all their slaves here, purchased for them a section of land, and even helped them to start the new life by furnishing cash for initial supplies.

The mother of one of the families died recently at the age of ninety-two. Her husband had died previously at the age of eighty-six. One of her sons recently brought her slave papers for me to see.

They are written in longhand as follows:

No. 243
Virginia: King William County, to-wit:
Registered in my office: Charlotte,
brown complexion, aged ten years, is
four feet and four inches high, has no
apparent mark or scar on her head, face
or hands and was emancipated by the last
will and testament of Ann. W. Taliafero,
deceased, which was duly recorded in the
clerk's office of King William County
Court on the 27th day of November 1854.
In testimony whereof, I have hereunto
set my hand as Clerk of the said
SEAL Court and affixed the seal of
said county this 27th day of August 1855.
W. Tollard, clk.

To Charlotte and her husband were born eight children, six boys, and two girls. Three have died, one of whom ran a successful dairy farm. Among the survivors are, one schoolteacher, one M.D., one dentist, one pharmacist, and one who lives here, badly crippled by a mine injury. As a family, they are intelligent, quiet, courteous, useful citizens.

One Sunday evening we drove to the country to make a call. It was a road new to me. We finally mounted a very steep hill so narrow that it would have been impossible to pass another car. The farm we were seeking was at the summit. I stood and beheld a new world of hilltops and trees and wondered if I had stumbled upon a Shangri-La.

A white paling fence surrounded the large yard. A beautiful old red brick house faced the road. It had fine proportions. The small-paned windows were clearly accented by sideburns of green shutters and by unthinned eyebrows of cut stone. Under a small portico was a beautiful doorway. A lovely old glass fan extended the full width of the eight-panel door and the glass sidelights.

I was warmly invited in by a friendly foreign voice at the gate. We entered the kitchen to find it bubbling with people, all chattering in an unfamiliar tongue. By a process of talking louder than the others and by frowning darkly at their continued efforts, the eldest woman finally monopolized the conversation to the exclusion of family, friends, and me.

"We buy this farm and pay cash moneys to man. My man he save money he make in mine. He hurt bad in mine. Don't git no compisation so we mus buy farm. We pay all our moneys for farm. When we come, no back door, lots windows out.
"We got no moneys left, not one dollars. Try git flour, chicken feed, middlins at store. No can git, because no money. Noting to eat tree days. (Rubbing stomach). We have trouble, trouble.
"Soon I start git baby. No have one for 18 years. I swell up my legs. I swell up my all over. (Many gestures.) I seeck [sick]. I paint and plaster house but seeck all time. (Mal de mer gestures). Man seeck but mus make food. Tree week too soon I start have baby. Make 7 quart water on floor. I say my son, 'Go queeck, git Doctor.' My son he run downhill tree mile. He git skin off hand pounding on. Doctor's door, no go. He run other Doctor's house, make skin off other hand he pound

so hard, no go. He start run home, stops car and say to neighbor, 'My mother die, you come car.'

"They come. I say, 'Take me hospital.' I go hospital have baby, big size baby. No got milk. I squeeze breasts (gestures) no drop milk. Baby no grow. Try eagle milk, I try men's (Mennen's I suppose) milk. Try everyting. Baby no eat. In hospital I git pain in my back side (gestures). Nurses say they no can put hot tings on back because doctors no say. I yell. I yell louder. I yell all time loud. They git hot water.

"I seeck all time, still yet seeck ole woman. Never be no better. (Shaking head dolefully)."

I began to wonder if Jerry would ever return, or if I would have to help bring the illnesses of 18 years up to date. I interrupted the flow of words for the first time.

"I think you will soon feel better. You don't look old. How old are you?"

"I ole woman, die someday soon may be. Be 46 my nex birtday."

Her four gold teeth beamed benignly, and the audience looked surprised when I mentioned that I liked the house.

The husband brightened, "I show heem to you."

There were six in the procession headed by husband with an oil lamp. When we reached the front hall with its lovely curving stairway and classic doorway, he stopped and said, "I pretty soon feex door. Put nize glass door some day pretty soon may be."

Sometimes I can't subdue my wide reforming streak. "But that door is really beautiful—just like the pictures in books. Do please leave it."

"You like heem? O.K., ladee, I leave heem may be." And I breathed a sigh of relief.

Every room in the house seemed at least eighteen feet square and each had its fireplace and slop jar—the latter had the spotlight. One room had three full-sized beds and several odd pieces and appeared unfurnished. The fireplaces were plastered up and large coal monstrosities were substituted. The fireplace in the kitchen was at least twelve feet wide. One beautiful bedroom with lovely old mantel, deep windowsills, long windows, and wide floorboards, contained a garish modernistic bedroom suite in several tones of light wood, and on the painfully modern blonde bed was a three-foot thick goose-down tick. All the beds in the house had these instead of covers.

During the tour, my original informant took off again, "Trouble, trouble, all time trouble. Lose six, one year." (I thought she meant children but discovered it was year old calves.) "Lose two horse. Both horse try have baby. One die. One break leg and my man shoot heem. My baby—no baby 18 year—get seecker. She die after other doctor leave twenty minutes. I seeck all time now."

A bright smile lighted her face as she forgot her ills long enough to say, "You come visit to us Lady. Stay maybe tree week. One ole man 82, he was leetle boy this house, he come stay tree week. Got catched in barb fence but not hurt none. Just got tore in the pantz. My leetle boy pull heem out."
I didn't want to take that chance, but I thanked her warmly and said I'd love a visit.

We have the poor with us. We have the W.P.A. in generous numbers. We also have the W.O.O. (without obvious occupation—past or present). Many of these have never been known to work. They drape themselves at various intersections near the center of the village and busy themselves with nothing more constructive than a process of gradually changing the color of the cement. How they keep so plentifully supplied with tobacco is a mystery.

Occasionally one drops from the ranks by death or a mild and temporary desire to work for a brief interlude but there is a long waiting list.

There are those in our town who would be social climbers if there were any place to climb and the ascent not too arduous. There are those who know their arts. One has impressed me by saying that she has a lampshade that, "That guy Rembran" painted. A literary light told me that her favorite English writer is Hugh Wallhide. There are those of us with aspirations, queen of whom is the mother of six who, with gold teeth, a droopy abdomen, a shuffling walk, a dirty body, and a filthy house, wants to be an interior decorator. And there are some with real talent who are completely submerged with large families, small houses, and no money.

Of churches, there are six for a population of about 1200. When the aid societies cook for the county fair, no good Presbyterian would be so base to betray the cash amount of business to their enemy Methodists and vice versa. Nor is the spy system effectual, but the food of both is excellent.

We have our little wars, our bickerings, our quarrels. We have the war of the taxed vs. the untaxed, the war of the undertakers, that of the political parties, and that of the union adherents vs. the non-union. The undercover war of the sexes reminds me of the remark of an elderly anti-suffrage gentleman, member of the school board, who resented a woman on the board with the graphic statement, "It just ain't no place for pink bloomers."

The school board has its disagreements internally and from without. It has been the exception to have board members with a background of formal education. Factions differ violently as to the qualifications of the teachers, superintendent, the various ministers, and public officials. Some want 6% beer and Sunday movies. More do not. The war of the generations goes on apace here as elsewhere. The Superintendent of Schools handed me this anonymous card the other day:

> Superdendent,
> We think it is a consern of the school that the good people of this town has to watch the school kids go along the street making love all day, it is a sore eye to look at. It is sicking to see the Bailey boy and the Beecher girl and others with there arms around each other and holding hands. It is a sicking sore eye and you should stop it. What do you get paid for?

The choirs fuss, the band mothers quarrel to the death, the quilting groups, the sewing societies, and rival bridge clubs gossip.

Many people do not enter public places to drink 3% beer or the like. This is unique enough to be seen refreshing to me which is probably a carryover from the days when, as children, we were told, "Pour the grape juice out of the bottle before you drink it, children." I still subconsciously associate bottles with sin.

Many civic-minded citizens keep farm animals in the city limits. The mayor has a cow. Pigs, horses, cows, and chickens are a part of many family circles. I know one family, just out of town, that lets the chickens and turkeys roost in the kitchen at night. I'd like a cow, but I can't honestly decide whether it is because I want milk for the family or manure for the roses.

There was one time when Jerry and I were in the country that we were offered a rickety cow on a bill. I offered to drive the car home and let him lead the cow. The scene is better described without the direct conversation. It didn't change his mind even when I suggested that he could carry his medical bag on the other hand so chance onlookers would not think he had changed occupations.

The neighbor's chickens are allowed two or three weeks of unadulterated freedom in the early spring at which time they descend on our yard in delirious delight and like whirling dervishes feast on all the little perennial seeds which would fill the vacant spots in the flower borders were Nature allowed to be kind. They have unallowed orgies at other intervals.

Progress comes slowly and is accepted as a last resort. Few really wanted city water which was recently made a reality. It was worked up as a state of mob psychology. Many still cling to the old ways. Nearly every backyard has its outside toilet. The pleasure of dining in the garden is somewhat dimmed by the knowledge of their existence. They are not the substantial, well painted and constructed models with small windows almost too small for openings of wren houses—

one of the concrete evidences of the success of the W.P.A.—but are weathered, faithful unpainted models depending on rear draft, open-door policy, and wide cracks for their air conditioning, with just an occasional star or new moon. I constantly marvel at the all-conclusive love of a paternal government that cannot only build these gigantic birdhouses but can furnish several thousand dollars to drain the quarter stretch of the county fairground which is used three days a year at a loss, many thousand for a football stadium in which are played about five games a year, many more thousands for the city water system, sufficient funds to repaint the school buildings, and apparently limitless amounts to encourage people of the right political faith to relinquish their accustomed lives of idleness.

Family life is much more complex than surface appearances would indicate. When small bits of gossip and scandal are so thoroughly worried along from one doorstep to another and never allowed to die, I shudder to think what would happen to town morale if all could see through the doctor's eyes. The foundations of home, school, and church would totter. But this will not happen for the secrets of attempted suicides, abortions, false parentage, acquired diseases are never disclosed. The questions of petty morals will still remain paramount and a few will always try to dominate the thinking of the many.

I would not sound too critical or unsympathetic. The neighbor who thinks short-haired dogs immodest, would be the first to do a neighborly deed. And the one who makes a calendar of all marriage dates and has even been known to juggle them a bit like chessmen would be the first to help with the care of an unwanted child. The mother who told me she knew why her little son died, "The Lord knew I had too much to do," took the best of care of Edward while he lived and was astonished when I asked, "If the Lord has your good at heart, why didn't he take you and let you rest and leave Edward, whose life was just beginning?"

We know a classic case where a man's illegitimate daughter married his wife's illegitimate son, and all is well.

There is great loyalty to the little town; sometimes I think it is in inverse proportion to the advantages offered. But I find the advantages legion. When trouble comes, the town arises as one man to help the sick or grief-stricken.

The people are neighborly, leisurely, innately honest and they mean to be kind. It is not everywhere that the telephone repairman would stop to fit together sections of his ladder and anchor the euonymus vine to the chimney. Nor is it everywhere that one finds such keen interest in small detail which I discovered when a small child said happily, "My mother says your fingernails look like a wolf's."

I like the little patches of vegetables behind most houses, the solitary clumps of rhubarb, the snarled old grapevines, the ivy on old brick walls. I like the quiet streets at night when the last stragglers have shambled home and the trees touch fingers over the deserted village streets. Sometimes the darkness seems crowded with loneliness as one or two solitary figures stand like specters, motionless, voiceless, dead. The winds in the trees cry with longing for something not there. Peace? Quiet? Voices and figures that are gone? I can forget the whispers of gossip when I hear the rustle of the trees and feel the peace of an understanding Nature envelop me. When there is time, there is room to see the sky, blue through lacy leaves in summer and dull gray through a delicate tracery of twigs in winter. The sun rises and sets through no film of smoke or fog. One can wander mentally across half a hundred lovely hills.

Cities are near but we can select what we would of them. In this, I realize that I have a wise and far-seeing guardian angel. I need not take on activities of city life which keep one's time, but not interest, entirely occupied. I like to play bridge, but a bridge luncheon a day would sear my soul. Activity as such does not interest me and I want to enjoy in retrospect some concrete evidence of hours well spent. Perhaps for this reason gardening has greater appeal for me than golf. I am more inspired by raindrops in the heart of lupine leaves or on the unfolding rose petals than I am by traffic jams.

And I like to know my neighbors. One little girl, aged three, accustomed to plaudits, drew a chair up to the bier of an elderly neighbor. Death baffled her. She sang a few bars of Jesus Loves Me and stopped to see if it had the usual effect. Finally, she finished the song, climbed down from the chair, and said, "She must be dead."

Another time I was gathering roses along the garden wall while a neighbor boy was trying to combine paper and sticks into the magic of a kite. The wind disrupted every effort. Finally, he stopped his work and stood up and addressed the universe, "For heaven's sake, God, can't you turn off that wind for five minutes? I got work to do too."

Another lad wandered through the hedge one other day when our yard contained an unreasonable amount of manure ready to be incorporated into rose beds. He involuntarily upped his small nose and asked in wonderment, "You don't mean to say you buy that stuff?"

Yes, I enjoy my garden. In the Spring, in less than a minute, I can be in an old-fashioned violet patch that makes one dream dreams. I've been there when a brief shower came up and was bathed in fragrance.

I like the county fair and the small local movie which brings pictures late but the hysteria of advertising is over so we know what pictures are probably worth seeing. I have greater interest in our local high school athletic teams than I do in major league baseball which I know is the admission of a narrow mind!

I like living where houses and cars are seldom locked and where horses jog along, passed by flying cars in the streets. One morning I was helping to lay stepping stones in the front yard and I saw a village waif, who would live in our slum if we had one, riding in an outmoded high buggy with a bewhiskered driver behind a senile white horse whose coat was adorned with liverish yellow patches, and the lad was hiding his face with a ragged sleeve, embarrassed at being seen in such an old fashioned conveyance. It brightened my entire day.

Nor have you lived until your own backyard produces all your fresh fruit from trees planted by your own hand. Corn from the market and corn fifteen minutes from the garden to the boiling pot are two very different foods. I defy you to diet if you whiff Nan's country butter or the hams we cured ourselves. Our house is constantly filled with flowers from our own garden. As I write, tulips and apple blossoms are in a pink peach blow vase on the dining table. Lilacs perfume the house and yard. Three large stone jars are massed with cherry blossoms.

After all, I guess I'll forget my village woes, and urge Jerry to suppress city aspirations—not that there's the slightest danger. He hasn't time to worry about it, and he loves being a country doctor.

Cornelia's Parents

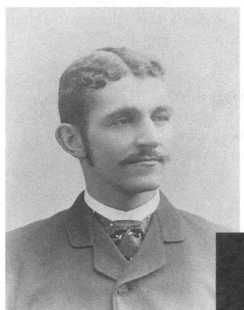

William Mahon Cattell
(1860-1931)

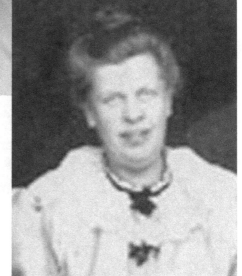

Edith Virginia Brenneman
(1864-1913)

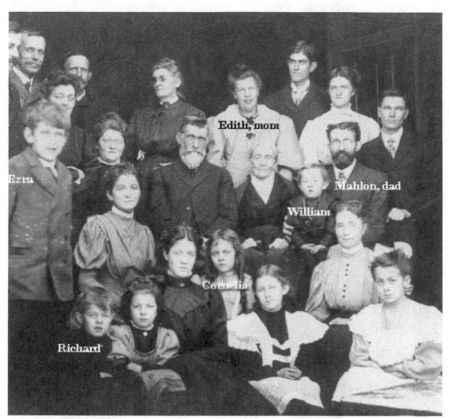

The Cattell family photo...man and woman behind Cornelia are
her grandfather and grandmother (in Quaker garb)

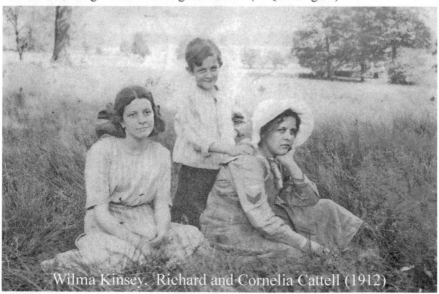

Wilma Kinsey, Richard and Cornelia Cattell (1912)

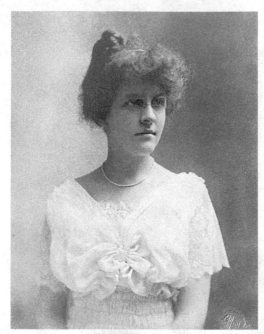

Cornelia at 18, c. 1918

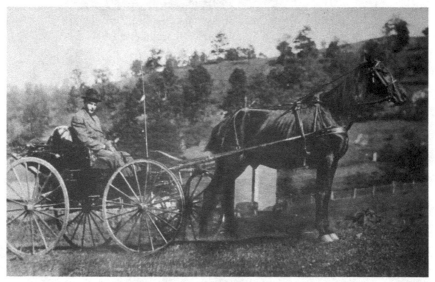

Young Dr. Jay Ira Thompson out for a house call c. 1920

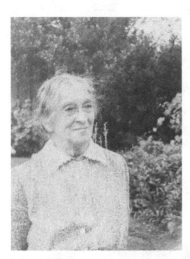

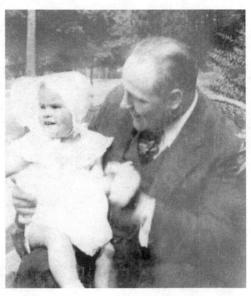

Aunt Lydia Cattell who lived
with them, c.1940

Doctor Jerry holding baby Nancy, c. 1919

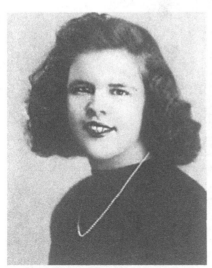

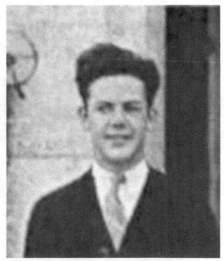

Daughter Nancy, high school
graduation photo, 1939

Howard Fisher, ward, high school
graduation photo, 1935

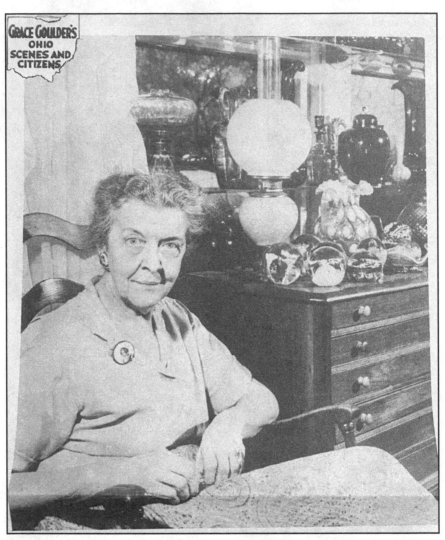

Cornelia feature in Cleveland *Plain Dealer* by Grace Goulder May 1962
(age 64). Titled:
"Mrs. Jerry Thompson, antique dealer and much else in Smithfield."

Quaker Life

[Cornelia's father, William Mahlon Cattell, came from a long line of Quakers. In 1893 he asked to be released from his Quaker church in order to marry Edith Virginia Brenneman, a non-Quaker. Marrying outside the faith was forbidden and was grounds for disownment. Seven years later in 1906, when William moved his family back to Mount Pleasant, Ohio, he and his family rejoined the Quaker church. Cornelia was brought up in the Quaker religion, but in later life did not attend meetings and baptized their daughter as Methodist.]

There are numerous descendants of the old Quaker families who were the town's first settlers. Their integrity is unquestioned. Their first Yearly Meeting in this section was held in nearby Mount Pleasant, in 1813 at which time their philosophy of religion was outlined and a code of discipline adopted. The women had a separate code until 1887. Many of their ideals, then and now, are an excellent standard to live by. In many ways their beliefs seem years ahead of the times. One of the fundamental aims is simplicity in all things—in habits, clothing, food, and customs such as marriage and burials. They urgently disapprove of the use of intoxicating beverages or tobacco.
The Discipline says:
"Friends are therefore tenderly, but most earnestly, admonished against its use, culture, manufacture, or traffic."

The older generation wore the plain clothes, both men and women. My grandmother was the last person in the church to wear the Quaker garb. The family has a number of Quaker outfits for old and young. Father kept a coat, adorned with worldly lapels, in town and changed when he left the boarding school for any reason as they were allowed nothing so modern there. The present Quakers, or Friends, do not follow the admonitions about dress so literally but they are instructed:

"We, therefore, urge our members that they teach diligently by precept, and exemplify by practice, true Christian simplicity in dress, and that moderation be observed in furnishing our houses and providing for our tables; that in all things, Friends may manifest in their habits, speech, and deportment that simplicity which the gospel enjoins."

I visited a Quaker boarding school to judge an oratorical contest and the evening meal consisted of cottage cheese, stewed tomatoes seasoned with cream and butter, fresh bread, honey, and whole milk for the beverage.

Their church services have no elaborate ritual, nor have marriages or burials. I attended a Friend's funeral when I was ten. We sat and sat and silently contemplated the virtues of the dead (or our overpowering desire for roller skates). At last, the minister stood. He wore a benign countenance and a rusty frock coat. He folded his hands and preached the funeral sermon. I quote it complete:

"When James Eldridge sold a quart of beans,
he sold a quart of beans."

The funeral was over.

The Discipline of the church further urges: "Friends are to avoid the custom of wearing or giving mourning habits, and all extravagant expense connected with the interment of the dead. They are admonished to avoid affixing expensive stones or monuments to graves."

Aunt Lydia says she thinks she will select her own modest funeral accessories and instead of flowers, which she loves, she wants the money sent to missions.

The Quaker marriage service is beautiful. After having received the permission of the church to marry, at the appointed time, the parties to be married stand, take each other by the hand, and declare audibly, "In the presence of the Lord and this assembly, I take to be my wife (or husband), promising with divine assistance, to be unto her (or him) a loving and faithful husband, (or wife) until death shall separate us." The guests sign the Quaker marriage certificate and the service is over. Promises are not made to a minister but with the knowledge and blessing of The Lord and The Meeting.

The beliefs concerning war and the care of the indigent are well known. War is a crime and cannot be countenanced by a sect that aims to "promote understanding and harmony between classes, races and political divisions of mankind."

The poor are to be cared for but must in turn heed the admonitions of the church as to how they can best help themselves. Friends are constantly urged to "frequently inspect the state of their affairs, and keep their accounts so clear and accurate that they may at any time easily know whether they are living within the bounds of circum- stances." (Shouldn't we all?) I still have my grandfather's day books in which accurate records of every cent spent or taken in is recorded.

Those "who have fallen short of paying their just debts, although they may have obtained a legal discharge by the voluntary act of their creditors, should not regard their moral obligation to pay such debts to have ceased. But if they should be favored in the future with the ability to meet then, they should offer to make a readjustment with their creditors; and Friends should be careful in regard to receiving contributions or bequests for benevolent purposes from such persons until the claims against them are discharged."

The Friends as a church feel a keen responsibility for the moral as well as spiritual welfare of their members. Offenders are dealt with "in the spirit of restoring love." In cases where the offender does not need the admonitions, they are disowned.

The church in this little town was torn wide open some years ago be- cause of a division in the ranks caused when the Discipline was taken literally and the dictates of active individual consciences led them to dismiss a prominent member on the charge of "lying and deceitful living."

Many families occupy the farm homes which their parents and grandparents held before them. I have a copy of the Articles of Agreement made by an elderly father who owned one of these homes. He had conquered the forest, established a pioneer home, and started ten sons and daughters on the good way of life. When he felt the ravages of old age approaching, he wished to be relieved of some of his more active farm duties and he wanted his beloved farm to remain in the possession of one of his sons so he drew up the following paper:

> **Articles of Agreement** entered into the sixteenth day of September in the year of our Lord one thousand eight hundred and twenty-four and between Jacob Welday Senr., and his son Isaac Welday. Jacob Welday for twelve hundred dollars, will sell son Isaac Welday, the farm that the said Jacob purchased of Bazeel Wells, containing 190 acres. And also all the personal property that Jacob Welday is in possession of at the present time.

> The said Isaac further agrees that he will keep Jacob and his wife all the remainder of their days in sufficiency of vitlings [food] and clothing and in case of sickness Isaac is to furnish Jacob and his wife with a suitable [diet] and that Isaac cannot sell or dispose of the farm or any part of it while Jacob and wife lives.

> And Jacob is to have his usual seat at the table and the rooms that he has usually slept in. Also Jacob is to have the arm chair to sit in and the bench behind the stove to lie on at any time that he may deem proper and Isaac will not allow any dancing or anything of that nature in the house while Jacob and wife, or either of them liveth. And he further agrees that he will furnish Jacob with a horse and saddle and bridle to ride where ,when, and often as Jacob may think proper.

> **Post script**: Isaac further agrees to mend and wash all the clothing and bedding in good order belonging to the said Jacob and Mary when needed.

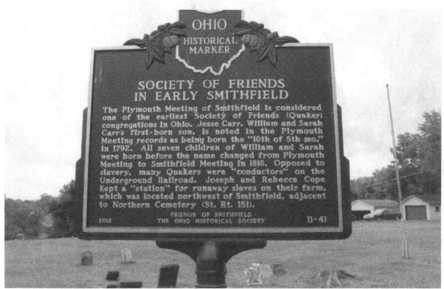

Marker at site of Quaker Yearly Meeting House in Smithfield

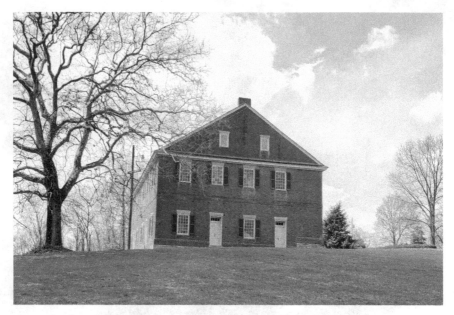

Quaker Yearly Meeting House in Mount Plesant, Ohio, also a center for anti-slavery writing and part of the Underground Railroad

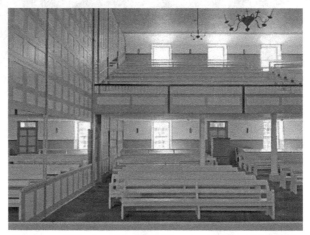

Interior of Quaker Meeting House at Mount Pleasant

We Acquire a Family

[Howard Fisher (b. 1918), the son of Lewis and Rachel Fisher, came to live with Cornelia and Jay Thompson in 1932 after the death of his father. His mother died nine years earlier leaving Lewis to raise five children. Though loved and cared for as an adopted son, the 1940 census referred to him as a 'ward' of the Thompson family.]

Housekeeping in the country doctor's household proved to be a hiccupy affair from the start. Our house was not completely finished for several months after our marriage, so we lived with Father. When it was finally ready, Jerry conveniently sprained his ankle and so was unable to do any of the actual moving.

The first two days in the new home were significant. It was well that I saw ahead as through a glass darkly. Everything looked fresh and very beautiful to my prejudiced eyes. I planned what I thought was a perfect dinner for the first evening. The table was lovely with our new silver, dishes, and linen. I had gathered many flowers from the garden which was too new to offer more than annuals. A bowl of pink snapdragons, blue Chinese forget-me-nots, and white baby's breath smiled in the center of the table.

That morning Jerry had said, "Let's forget sick babies, broken bones, accidents, diarrhea, babies due, and just sit and enjoy this day. After all, it's the first day in our new home." He had gone out before noon, so I expected him momentarily.

A man, who stuttered so badly that I could not understand his errand, waited in the living room for over an hour. His affliction was so pronounced that I wasn't even sure he wanted Jerry. I'm no help to a stutterer. I have a mad desire to bridge the gaps and so suggest one wrong word after another. This causes both the stutterer, and the would-be little helper, to flush with embarrassment. Jerry handles them better. He lights as many cigarettes as necessary and waits so long that I want to fill the great open spaces with lengthy screams, or at least yodels.

I lighted the candles at 6:30. I unlighted them at 7:30. Still no Jerry.

During early evening a patient came who was having terrible muscular spasms in his legs due to a bad injury in the mines. He sat twitching in agony. The callers, telephone, and doorbell kept me from any sustained interest in reading. About 10:30 a patient came who asked if she might wait for the doctor as she lived some distance away and was suffering from intense abdominal pain. I made her welcome and occupied my hands with knitting while my first two callers and I followed a fine story of hers that I have always wished had been my own experience.

Visiting in a strange house for the first time, she said she sat in the kitchen watching her hostess prepare dinner. On a chair beside her sat a huge white cat with abnormally large green eyes. She was fascinated by the penetrating gaze of the green eyes but chatted with her hostess. She wore a wristwatch and just happened to notice that the cat sat without moving or averting its gaze, for twenty-five minutes. There were only two doors into the room, both of which were closed, and she sat between the cat and the doors. Suddenly the cat was no longer there. She was startled and spoke,
"Where did your cat go?"
No door had opened. "Cat? We have no cat."
The reply amazed her, so she described the white cat minutely. Her hostess smiled.
"Oh, yes, that cat. Everybody sees that cat here. We rent this house cheaply because no one else will live here. But we have no cat and there are none near."

My caller was not convinced, so she spent an hour hunting for the snow-white cat. Her hostess elaborated. "I have three clocks and I have never wound one since I came and that was two years ago. Do not be afraid. I like this ghost. It unlocks my bedroom door every night and often shakes my bed in passing, but I am not afraid because I believe it is friendly."

The patient who stuttered forgot himself to say, "Some cat!" The man with the terrible pain in his legs had for a moment forgotten his pain, and I nearly forgot that I had been waiting eleven hours for Jerry.

The patient finally ran out of conversation, grew weary of waiting, and so took her abdominal pain and went home. The others followed suit. Her tale had interested but not soothed me.

At midnight, I fell asleep exhausted from my role as country doctor's wife and housekeeper. I was not then geared to disappointment as I am now. I have learned to count on not going, then it is a gorgeous surprise if we do. Shortly after daylight, I hurried downstairs and prepared the perfect breakfast. Waited. NO Jerry. When he, at last, came home at 1. P.M., there was no lunch on the table.

In spite of the unpropitious beginning, the days were happy ones, although they continued to defy any efforts to plan a scheme for living. Jerry was always busy, and I found many interests. Gardening was a great delight even though the phone always rang when I was on my knees in the farthest corner of the garden. I was still in the delicious state of ignorance that knew nothing of black spot, black beetle, tent caterpillars, aster wilt, dahlia borers, oyster scale, aphis, early frosts, brown patch, neighbor's dogs and children, anthracnose, and dictator plants, (like physostegia, Chinese lantern, veronica, cosmos, which reach out without conscience and seize ground reserved for quiet pansy faces). I unconsciously believed that if I tucked in a seed or lovingly set a plant or bulb or bush, it would flourish forever, making me an integrated part of creation. It was not long before I began to wonder why in heaven's name we had built on property without trees. The country and no trees! Now, however, I feel like Nature's first assistant because we are responsible for every tree, plant, and grass blade. Our own Chinese elm towers many feet in the air and its feathery branches rejoice when our wren families leave their tiny houses to sing exultantly in its branches, unconscious of me except as a part of the garden. Tall silver maples cradle the neat nests of goldfinches whose wings flash gold in the sunlight. Two large cherry trees give generously of their fruit and blossoms as do many varieties of peach trees. A weathered apple tree makes the family a happier one because of its breathlessly lovely blossoms and its excellent fruit. They are all a source of unending delight to young climbers.

I haven't forgotten one of the early stages in gardening when Jerry went out to do his bit by hoeing. At that moment I was busy and did not go with him, but since then I have tactfully managed to accompany him on his rare spasms of garden work. It does not require much of my time. When I did go out, I was greeted by, "Where in creation did all these weeds come from? Look at all the burdocks I've chopped out." I looked at the wilted heap. They were the precious hollyhocks that I had started from seed and raised on the bottle. For just a second, I wondered if I really loved him.

Soon I had quite a large class in piano study. This paid fine dividends in satisfaction but certainly not in cash, for many failed to pay for lessons and music, and the yearly recital was expensive.

Substitute teaching in the high school was interesting even though I would dash up about 9 A.M. without any advance notice and attempt to teach any subject in the curriculum from languages and the classics to physics, chemistry, and mathematics without preparation. I was once taken by surprise to learn that a senior group thought Edgar Guest was the greatest living poet, Temple Bailey, and Kathleen Norris the greatest living women writers, and Zane Gray and Harold Bell Wright the finest writers among the men. Many of these children never go beyond high school. The tremendous responsibility for their future always weighs me down when I am teaching. I doubt if Beowulf and Chaucer will have lasting benefits for them.

For some time, I studied organ, played the small organ in one of the churches, and tried to improve the choir work. I was amused when a clacking tongue remarked in the village that, "Anyone can see the way she sits at the organ that she's expectin'." I wondered if I should have concentrated on the harp.

My choicest memory of my local squashed-in-the-bud concert career is the time I sang two numbers (rather well for me) at the local Farmer's Institute. When I had finished, the finesse lacking chairman rose, rubbed his palms together with relish, and said, "Now, we always save the best till last. The McGrew sisters will now sing." I heard my Father's amused chuckle several rows back.

My most unique undertaking was the establishment of a small circulating library. Even writing the word makes me laugh aloud. I had the mistaken idea that the reason the town didn't read—there may have been a solitary exception—was because it was expensive to buy books and there was no library. Books and magazines were my greatest extravagance, so I decided to offer to lend mine. I had cards printed, bought many new books, and waited. I'm still waiting and that was ten years ago. Only two people asked for books. I use the cards for recipes and for bridge scores and maybe someday I'll paper a hallway in the paper covers which says, "Circulating Library."

I should have known better because the previous winter I had persuaded a group of about twelve or fifteen people to buy a book each, thus enabling all of us to read that many new books. It was not entirely an unselfish scheme. I made the selections and arranged the purchase. It was NOT a successful venture. One husband was indignant to find his wife reading Hugh Walpole's corrupt *Winter's Moon* and hasn't had any respect for me since. Another nearly had a stroke over Eugene O'Niel's *Strange Interlude*. I offered to buy them back. The venture died a quick death.

The town now has a small branch of the Carnegie Library which is a hopeful project thanks to more W.P.A. money. It also boasts of a circulating library. The titles of the books in the latter fascinate me.

If these are lent, then it occurs to me, belatedly, that my effort did not sufficiently appeal to the baser nature of man.

For some time I managed without hiring help, but that meant that I was not only tied to the telephone but was alone many nights. On one such night when I was alone, and did not want to be, the doorbell rang at 2 A.M. Before I could get to the door, someone started pounding and shaking it. The dog and I peered out the front door to see who was trying to jar it from the hinges. I opened the door and, in a voice thick with excitement, a nondescript foreign accent, and a highly scented stimulant, he begged for a doctor. "Please, Lady, we need him right away." I explained that he was not in and that I did not know when to expect him. "My God, then I'm afraid he's done in. Toney's in the car, and you know he's been shot seven times before this. He's bleedin' sompin' awful and we're beinz followed."

I asked him to wait for a minute while I phoned to see if I could locate another doctor. It was not soothing when he followed me to the phone, tugging at my sleeve and urging me to hurry. No luck at the phone, so I told him to bring Toney in. I hastily spread a cover on the day bed and Toney was deposited on it. There was a greenish cast to his features, so I supposed he was in shock. I loosened his coat and discovered a ragged hole in his neck with blood gushing from it. What I supposed was the jugular vein was lying exposed and throbbing. All I knew to do was to try to get him warm and pray for Jerry's return. I attached two heating pads and found two hot water bottles which I hastily filled. When I returned, there was a pool of blood on the rug and down the side of the slipcover were dull red stains. I giddily thought that it clashed with the color scheme of the room like the covers of *Atlantic Monthly* and *Harper's* did with the several [garden] plans, but one cannot live on garden magazines alone. Perhaps, I mused, under the circumstances, it would be better for the doctor's wife to include a rusty red in future plans. Heat was beginning to restore him to consciousness when I heard the welcome screech of the brakes on our car.

It was after this incident that Jerry decided we must hire help, so the trial and error system was begun. Maid trouble is not one of my main subjects of conversation. While lengthy and heated discussions on the subject go on apace, I try to keep still. Sometimes I enjoy speculating on what would happen if the subject were banned at bridge parties and like gatherings. Personally, I'm more interested in what is being written or the happenings on the complicated political horizon but these trials, and the fate of world Jewry and the Dictatorships, are smothered by the paramount facts that Mary never even sees dust and dirty curtains, and her pie crusts are always tough. She insists on Thursday afternoon off, and "I know she was planning to ask for another raise."

I have enjoyed my hired girls, and even the so-called gardeners, who tell me they know I don't want the onions saved and I discover tulip bulbs in the trash. The community boasts of no skilled help, so we begin at scratch. This has some disadvantages as it is difficult to anticipate situations that arise. For example, I had never thought to ask Solomon not to sit in the rose arbor in the early evening trimming corns with a long knife while he sniffed the fragrance of roses and honeysuckle while I showed guests through the garden.

I take a middle road between the attitude of [Ralph Waldo Emerson] Emerson's wife, Lillian, who said that when she gave an order or new direction in the kitchen, she felt like a boy who threw a stone and ran, and that of some of my fellow townspeople who welcome them into the bosom of the family. I try to be reasonable, but I do not always give them all the white meat of the chicken as Father used to do with our housekeeper Lizzie. She ate at the table with us, and was served after Mother and Auntie, before the famished children. The following conversation always took place on Sundays when we had one chicken.

Father, "What piece would you like, Lizzie?"
Lizzie, "Well, I'll take the white meat if nobody else wants it."

We fed our chickens well, but if you will divide one—even a large stewed one with lots of gravy—among two parents, one aunt, one hired girl, five children, and usually company, you will understand how I felt. I yearned for plenty of white meat. She also rushed to defend her goal post, the cookie jar, every time she heard one of our ten small shoes. There was no armed neutrality between her and my four brothers. It was open warfare and their battles were mine. After those vain yearnings, it has seemed more good fortune than I deserve to have married a man who prefers the dark meat, and easy access to the cookie jar still seems marvelous.

My first help left indignantly because she could not eat with the family. I later learned that it was village custom to treat the hired help as members of the family.

My second was young when she came. She stayed several years and went to school. I was genuinely interested in the child, made all her clothes, and tried in general to aid her. For a time I tried to help her with her school work but stopped after an hour spent on the history of Ohio when she told me in reviewing that Coolidge was the capital. She loved to watch Nancy read her encyclopedia, and she did her daily rounds with a 'whip and a smack'. March, to her, came in like a lion and went out like a sheep.

Missing her one day, I found her conducting a robin funeral. A neighboring scooter was the hearse. She read from Moses and Aaron, omitting any difficult words. She did all the mourning, wailing loud and long. The flower arrangements bore the inscriptions:

Hour Darling
God Bless Our Bird
With Love From The Loge

To get first-hand information of Life after Death, she buried her doll and dug it up every day or so to study results. She had a sunny disposition and learned to do everything my way, from cooking to arranging flowers, but in a few years, she developed aspirations, business and social and has now left.

I was glad to have help in the house when our Nancy arrived four years after we were married. Her arrival had been anticipated for four long years by many overactive imaginations, so the interest had waned for all but us. I had contracted whooping cough from a patient of Jerry's. I remember an amusing incident shortly before she came. A caller and I were having tea by the fire to the accompaniment of vigorous whoops. I volunteered, "I'm having a baby very soon."

This surprised her as my figure appeared normal. Her surprise was echoed by mine when she shook her head seriously and remarked, "Now, if you just live through it, it will be so nice for the doctor." I swallowed hard. "Yes, I think so too."

I did.

Family affairs moved along in the usual hectic fashion for three years. I had been much interested in Howard, a young boy who delivered our papers. I was first attracted to him because he looked like my brothers at that age. His mother had died when he was five and the Father had made a valiant effort to keep the family intact. When his father died suddenly one day late in May, we asked for Howard. Two younger sisters were to go to a government home for soldier's orphans. The older ones could take care of themselves. Howard was then eleven and completing the eighth grade with excellent marks in his studies. I learned after he came that he sat in the back row at the grade school commencement because his graduation clothes consisted of a heavy black sweater which had belonged to one of his older brothers and which he had turned wrong side out so the yellow school letter wouldn't show and his only trousers whose frayed bottoms he trimmed with scissors.

I believe it is less of a problem to take an older child into the family than it is to take a baby. The child does not need to pass through an inevitable emotional period of wondering about his parents. Even in the happiest adoptions, I cannot imagine not wondering about one's heritage. And the life pattern of the older child has been fairly well set.

In every sense, we look on him as a son, but in addition, we have a closer relationship as we are more in sympathy than most parents and children, and we share the viewpoint of the same generation. Surely, a son of our own could be no greater joy or satisfaction.

There were adjustments to make in family plans. Howard had been here less than a week when Jerry and I realized that Nancy was not feeling as well as usual. It proved to be endocarditis, a heart condition, and she was put to bed for an indefinite time. Before a week had passed, I received a long-distance call saying that Aunt Lydia was very ill and could we come and get her. She had been staying with relatives for a time but had gone to the hospital suffering from a general physical breakdown. After Nancy was asleep that evening, we drove sixty miles to the hospital where we found Aunt Lydia, my father's single sister, in bad physical condition and weighing less than 90 pounds. Jerry picked her up like a baby and laid her in the back seat. For months she and Nancy were bedfast. Jerry would carry them out to cots in the backyard on good days. The rest and care restored them to perfect health, but it was an uneasy period for all of us.

Our Nancy [1928-1983] is now completing grade five. According to one who helps us occasionally, she is a mannerable child. She has not seemed to need much of "the treatment that grows on trees," quoting the same authority. I am happy that she has a good disposition and a keen sense of humor. I'm entranced with her vocabulary. We were playing a guessing game the other night on the porch and I suggested the initials F.V. (flower vase). Instantly she mentioned Forsythia Vine, Fan Vibration, Flower Vegetation, Figtitious Varieties. When we asked her what she wanted for Christmas she said, "I have just one urgency—a great urgency—for a Princess Elizabeth doll." She occasionally speaks like her father's child. I called one day to ask what she was doing and she replied, "I'm taking care of the waste accumulation in my nose."

When she was six, I found her propped up in bed with a book of Thornton Wilder's on her knees. She looked up at me with a quizzical expression. "This is the third time I've tried to read *Heaven's Desperation*. What do you like about it?"

She no longer thinks that the things in the front of her head, such as the poems "Trees" and "The Night before Christmas" will fall back if she turns on her back in bed. She hopes Joe Penner [radio and film comedian] will never be out of fame on the radio. Looking at a catalog of fruit trees, she exclaimed, "My, how these do appetize me." Recently she began work on Anton Rubinstein's "Angelic Dream" in her piano work with me. There is much repetition of chords, which is the reason I had selected it. After reading it through, she remarked, "Poor Anthony, I guess he wasn't familiar with many chords. Or maybe he just got tired too soon at the piano, like I do." She thinks her Daddy should concentrate his efforts on finding a serum for hiccoughs. When I recently suggested that she eat a bunch of our fine grapes, which are so plentiful and so beautiful that I keep tall old glass dishes filled to overflowing, she interrupted the process to remark, "If you can believe it, the very first one was abscessed."

Our Howard is finishing college this year. He has happily held part-time jobs which have helped with his expenses. Nancy wrote one of her uncles saying, "Howy would love to come to your wedding but he scrubs at Ohio University." He and his schoolmates have a sound sense of values. His trips to and from college have been interesting experiences as he insists on thumbing. I urge him to write down some of the more interesting ones. The last trip back brought this account of it by mail:

IS COLLEGE WORTH IT?
A Tragi-Comedy in Five Acts.
By Howard

Prologue
Q:—How long does it take you to get to school, Howard?
A—About six hours.
Q—How long do you have to wait for rides?
A—Usually about twenty minutes.

Act 1.

Scene 1.

Time: 10:30 A.M. Place: The western edge of a country town on U.S. Route 22.

A medium-sized young man is forlornly waving to occupants of eastbound autos, said occupants going who knows where, said young man, desiring an education, trying to thumb his way to college. Our hero's family have just left him standing along the roadside, traveling case in hand, raincoat thrown over his shoulder.

Scene 2.

Time: 12:15 P.M.

Place: Same.

Act II.

Scene 1.

Time: 1 P.M.

Place: Small town, a supposedly thriving junior city, 20 miles from place in Act 1, Scene 1.

Our hero is in high spirits, contemplating an early arrival at his destination, now only 110 miles farther.

Scene 3.

Time 5:30 P.M.

Place: Same 20 miles from Act 1.

The aforementioned hero has seen most of the small town's 5000 inhabitants, including numerous and friendly young ladies, but has decided that in four hours one can see enough beauty to last a lifetime. Right now he is concerned with neither beauty nor lifetimes. College remains the same 110 miles away. HERO YAWNS.

Act III.

Scene 1.

Time: 7:00 P.M.

Place: Small city 65 miles from Act II. Town boasts many pretty young girls but apparently, no automobiles with empty seats or social conscience ever leaves city after dusk. At the end of 24 hours, hero is tired, no longer feels able to wave at pretty girls or passing motorists. Here he meets another college-bound thumb-er and they gird themselves for a 55-mile leap into the wilderness. For it is here they leave well-traveled Route 22 and head South into the great darkness.

Scene 2.
Time: 9:30 PM.
Place: Same City. Hero has become quite chummy with his co-adventurer. TWO persons cannot stand side by side for 24 hours waving hopefully at tens of thousands of passing motorists without revealing to each other most of their past histories.

Act IV.
Scene 1.
Time 11 P.M.
Place: Small town, 7 houses, a gas station, a grocery store, all dark. 11 miles from college. Only a devilish Fate, reserved for hitchhikers, could have made a night so dark! An unsympathetic motorist let us out here because he lived here—only God knows why. Our actors had no alternative but to start to walk.

Scene 2.
Time 11:30 P.M.
Place: 2 1/2 miles along road, all 2 1/2 accomplished by leg action. An unwary farmer, who should have known better than to pick up two disheveled unknowns (we no longer looked like college material) at that time of night, stops, takes boys to city, proves his true value to his country by delivering boys to their respective doorsteps. Whatta man!

Act V.
Scene 1.
Time: midnight
Place: Bedroom. All that can be seen of our hero is a mop of curly black hair, slightly grayed from dust. Morpheus, man's only true friend, holds him in his soothing arms.

Curtain

When Howard first came, he was voluntarily helping me with the dishes one evening. He chuckled and said, "This amuses me. On my eleventh birthday, I got up in the morning and announced to my father and my sisters, 'No more dishes. I am now a man and will not do woman's work.' And the funny thing is that I got away with it."

I asked him if he knew what he wanted to do when he grew up. He did. "Well, I figure by that time, Babe Ruth will be through." He no longer aspires to be Babe's successor and peer. He will be satisfied if he can tell U. S. Steel or Mr. Morganthau [Secretary of the Treasury under Roosevelt] where they are slipping. The intricacies of business hold his interest. He tried pre-medics for a year before we discovered that he hated it and only did it because he thought it would please Jerry.

Aunt Lydia is eighty-two, mentally alert, and physically well, though not strong. She has not strayed an inch from the early strict Quaker teaching. She would not dream of attending a movie, feeling sure, from hearsay, not experience, that they are all harmful in influence. Sunday papers would never be purchased by her, but she is alert to world affairs, so asks us on Sundays, "What did Hitler say?" or "What is the strike news?"

She worried for a week because she thought Jack Benny's radio take-off on Snow White, called "Snow White and the Seven Gangsters," was the original which we had considered a fine production. I try to cull magazines and call her attention to articles she would like. I know she reads many with one eye figuratively closed.

On her eighty-second birthday, we planned an open house and other pleasant features for the day. She was at breakfast when our foreign-born grocer arrived. I said, "Aunt Lydia is eighty-two today." He came into the dining room beaming, went over and gave her a resounding smack on the shoulder which nearly knocked her off her chair, and said, "Well, who'd have guessed you were such an old lady?" I choked on my coffee. I'd just as soon have slapped Queen Mary and shouted, "How's tricks, old girl!"

We had friends to tea, and in one of her small gifts was a card which she handed me to read. It said, "May you be happy today to prepare you for your birthday in Heaven." We both chuckled and she quietly said, "I am expecting to get there eventually, but I do not feel there is any hurry about it."

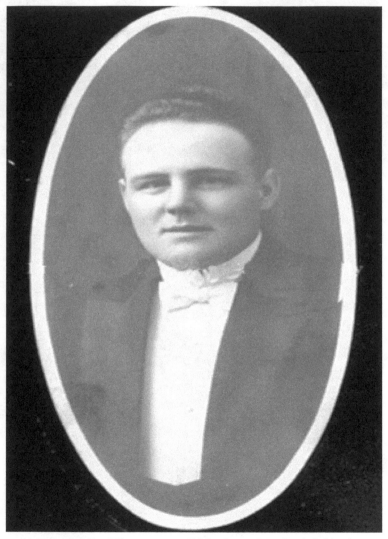

Dr. Jay Ira Thompson, Ohio State Medical School
graduation1914

One Monday

[Miss Mehitable MacGregor, Nancy's Scottish terrier was a gift from Cornelia's brother Dr Richard Cattell. He was a famous doctor in his time having Sir Anthony Eden, then Great Britain's foreign secretary, later Prime Minister, as a patient. In a letter to Cornelia, Richard states, "Mr. Eden is 11 days post-op and very well, a delightful person. He and Mrs. Eden will dine with us at home next Sunday."]

Lucius Beebe in a recent issue of *You* says that women have more time to devote to perfecting their persons than men. I wonder. Things have happened to my time in the course of busy days. Recently, reverberations from a depression led me to think that I should do without a maid. I had temporarily forgotten that there are only twenty-four hours in a day (we need at least sixty), while I was impressed by hearing a very close member of the family say that doing one's own work adds dignity to the stature. The soul wasn't mentioned, the family purse was.

I began with high courage by reducing the family payroll. Tactfully, I dismissed Zelda who had a doll in her room named Tranquillidor. She perched the coffee, unattached the iron, and apparently greased the dishpan. On a recent night, she had met us at the door smiling, "Boy, was there an accident while you were gone! They were all cut up, and drunk. I knew where you were, but I hated to call you, so I just fixed them all up myself, and sent them home. You won't even need to see them, Doctor."

It was easy to face the prospect of the separation. I became solo director and producer. I chased my tail so many hours a day I wished

I knew how Mr. Edison had managed on a four-hour sleep average. By evening I was emotionally and physically at low ebb. I would grit my teeth, and murmur to myself, "This is the end, not another day. I'll hire two maids." But morning found me fresh with hope, and I stuck out my neck again, and yet again. Jerry thought I loved it, which proves Hitler's premise in *Mein Kampf* that with propaganda one can do anything, and also that large lies are easier to believe than small ones.

Monday was an average day during my self-inflicted servitude. A glorious sunrise awoke me—I do not leap up to greet the dawn like one I read about, eager to begin setting up exercises or to have a morning canter. We had probably retired about two AM, if we weren't up all night, and answered the phone or door twice between then, and dawn, so I gave myself a push, and arose half-conscious, dabbled in a little water, swathed myself in a dressing gown, laid out Nancy's clothes, and checked to see that she was up, and washing.

This particular morning Nancy, with great excitement, drew out the first name from a box of wedding cake she had slept on.* The result did not please her.

"But I can't have Nelson Eddy [singer, and actor] come out first. I want him to be the last, so I'll just put him in again, and mix them up."

I cantered down to begin my day. It was a cool fall morning, and Solomon [Byers] had a blazing fire in the living room grate and had water on for coffee. He is the family handyman and mascot whom we acquired as a legacy from the social service. As I started the Silex, put out the milk bottles, set a table by the fire, and hurried with breakfast, I pondered on some of his qualifications, and eccentricities.

He not only thinks he can do everything, but there really are a great many things he can do. At first, he thought I was too young to know how to do anything, but recently he spoke with a hush in his voice, "Miss, you've learned me somepin'. I never knowed a lady could work." He is never tired, and never out of humor. When I hired him, he tried to present a true picture of himself, "Miss, I has only one vice. I likes to play the numbers. A man was to have somepin' to think about when it isn't womin."

He has been here a long time. The doorbell interrupted my thoughts. My heart lurched when I saw a mangey horse standing at the curb. He wasn't even enjoying his adventure in the city. A dark mountain of flesh stood at the door. He looked larger than the horse, and almost as mangey. Tears were streaming down his face. If I hadn't seen this before, I'd probably have wept with him, but I had learned my lesson by asking him to wait for the doctor one winter night, and we sat until 3 A.M. sharing his misery. It is impossible to reach his place by car, so he uses tears at will to detract from the walk necessary, and the large balance on the books.

I took for granted that his wife was dying again and assured him that the doctor would come. He went off comforted, a broad smile breaking through the simulated gloom, and I felt sure he would be carrying that horse before he reached home.

When Nancy came down to have her hair brushed, she found her breakfast ready by the fire. I queried, "Would you like a piece of coffee cake?"
"Oh, yes, please, I have a large compassion for some."

He chatted while she ate, and I had my coffee. With two cups of good coffee, I was in a suitable frame of mind to face the day with its uncertain vicissitudes. After twenty minutes of supervised practice, I saw Nancy off to school.

While Jerry ate, I had had another cup of coffee with him. Afterward, I gathered up the faded flowers and scattered newspapers, dusted the living room, and ran the vacuum.
The doorbell interrupted the latter. I opened the door to find a small neighbor child smiling at me.
"Is Nancy at home?"

"No, dear, she's at school now."
There was another smile, then, "I thought she would be."

Breakfast installments continued. Lydia came next, and while she ate,
I prepared breakfast for Solomon and our laundryman, in the kitchen.
Solomon's food is an easy matter. Any food pleases him if it is greasy.
The ultimate in praise is "It et good" or "it drunk good." I know it
is just fair in his grease-minded opinion if he says, "s'all right, Miss."
Solomon expects to live forever. "Miss, when I'm old I won't know
whether it's because my Insides is preserved in alcohol or grease. Both
is healthy, and I've had lots of both."

The laundryman is well named, Pleasant Smith. He doesn't care what
the food is just so there is enough. He has pernicious anemia, and an
eye for women. He has washed for us for years in return for the necessary liver extract plus donations of one sort or another.

This Monday morning I longed to add a little ground glass to his
breakfast, as the previous wash day he had boiled a black sock with
the white clothes, and had spilled chlorox on a white silk dress leaving it in great holes. He wears contrition as an easy cloak and finds it
less of a nuisance to be smilingly contrite than to be careful enough
to avoid disaster. He has no money, but has a willing and cheerful
disposition. That morning he brought the news that he knew where
we could buy a fine pony for Nancy. Said pony could trot, single-foot,
and cantaloupe. I decided to let him live.

After snatching the dishes from the table so that Solomon could wash
them, I made starch and cooked an evil-looking mixture for Hitty,
and her cavernous puppies. Hitty is Nancy's Scottish terrier named
Miss Mehitable MacGregor. There have been times when the care of
Mehitable has been a little trying. At such times Nancy refers to her
as being hot. When I wrote Howard that Nancy stood in front of the
kennel—Jail—saying to Hot Hitty, "Don't worry, Honey. Pretty soon
you'll be cooled off, and can come home," Howard's answer was,

 Hot,
 Hitty hot?
 What?

Hitty not hot?
Good for Hitty,
Frisky, and pretty.
Isn't it a pity
This can't be a ditty?
Why not? (apologies to Gertrude [Gertrude Stein])

But the fact remains that she is of noble lineage. Her puppies, due to insecure fencing, are 50% less noble, Isaiah, Jeremiah, Lamentations, and Ezekiel. Let no one suppose Nancy's two weeks in summer bible school left no imprint. Ezekiel is Nancy's favorite, but she has promised her to Solomon for his grand baby.

Up to this point in the day, no hysteria, just speed, and super control. Upstairs I dashed, bathed, dressed, gathered up the tag ends of the washing, and sorted out the things I would have to wash. Pleasant has no proper respect for silks and fine linen.

I hastily smoothed up the beds with a vow to do better the next time and smiled skeptically to myself when I remembered that one of my friends insists that her beds be stripped to the skin each day, and mattresses turned. The thought made me want to do a Mephistopheles from Faust where he sings, Ha, Ha, Ha's in three octaves. The dust mop and I cavorted about where it would show the most. I cleaned shaving-lather off the lavatory in the bathroom and valeted for the entire family, more or less, snorting probably, but I don't remember. When Jerry's mother visits us, and sees his clothes on the floor, she gets a faraway look in her eye, and murmurs, "He was such a good boy, never any trouble." It is the logical place for the bromidic, Them Days Is Gone Forever, but I smile understandingly, and try to look dewey, feeling more like the Tammany Tiger.

I clutched the washing to my panting bosom and started for the laundry in the basement. Aunt Lydia's voice stopped me short. "I have finished darning the socks, and am putting a few stitches in Aunt Jane's Coverlet. Wouldn't this be a good day to wash it?"

Great Aunt Jane's coverlet had just come to light after years of storage, but I assured her that this was the day, and held it with my chin as I started down again. I tried to remember who it was that urged us not to build a clothes chute because of the danger of thieves. I would welcome a good sincere thief occasionally if it saved all the extra trips to the laundry. Just as well that I couldn't remember the identity of that well-intentioned friend, or the anti-backstairs advocate or the one-bathroom propagandist either.

The doorbell rang shrilly, and I dropped my pack to answer it. A smiling ebony face greeted me. With a generous flourish, he proffered me a bottle of vinegar-colored fluid, saying smilingly, "Don't spill it, Missus."

He wanted medicine to cure the symptoms as per said bottle and the note he brought. Jerry handed me the note as he exited to the office, keeping a straight face with difficulty.

> NOTE:
> (condishuns of Mary)
> Num Face
> Week Arms
> Stif Knees
> Soar in pam of hand, and stif.
> Stif, and sort of bownd feeling.
> Side pain in neck. Bouls tite. Jumping in rist.
> Feet num, and itchy in ball.

On to my washing, including the Rip Van Winkle coverlet. We have had city water for only one year, so I remembered to be thankful when I turned on the water. I still feel like a hussy every time I draw a tub half full of water for a bath. In the past, the water came from cisterns and wells. We then bathed in water the depth of which would never have inspired Archimedes. A loud knocking on the back door called me up from the laundry. I found a hungry elderly man who asked for something to eat. When I asked him in, he said he preferred to sit on the back steps in the sun as he was not clean enough to come in. I hastily filled a tray with a large serving of hash, six slices of bread, a plate of butter, and jelly, a pitcher of hot tea, a piece of stale cake, and a sack of candy that the family spurned. His eyes made me ashamed of my extra pounds. Not even a crumb was left on the tray. I questioned him, "Why don't you find regular work?" "Well, you see, Lady, I sailed for 26 years, and it ain't no way to prepare for hard times when you are old. I kint git no work." "How about the W.P.A?" "Well, you see, Lady, I ain't got what you'd call a legal place of res-I-dence ezactly so they won't give me no job. I see now that I'd be better off if I'd worked for one boss for forty or fifty years. Then you gotta chance. Goodbye, Lady, and thanks to ye."

He shambled down the steps, and I scurried back to the laundry. I stopped to ask Solomon to scrub down the back porch, but he professed to an attack of Flying Rheumatism. Flying anything had my sympathy just then—we compromised on gardening.

From the laundry I hurried to my desk to write a letter. I also took a minute to cross out a few items on a list of Things-We-Have-To-Have. This was the fifth re-write. I try to keep the list from becoming concrete until the need is past.

While Solomon was gone for the mail, I prepared things for lunch, and dinner: pared potatoes, and onions for French frying, scraped carrots, made a dessert, and cut some slices of country ham. Solomon was soon back, and I scanned the mail. Howard's laundry came from school late so I would have to wash it. In the empty cake box, I found a large sheet of paper inscribed More Please, and signed by six boys in his group at school. Another letter interested me when Jerry handed it to me later. It was unsigned, and read as follows:

Daer Dock Thompon, Sir, I bet you think I am a liar, but honest I have enuf truble to drive me nuts, mother in hospital, sister died, and while we was away the Boy got sick to his stomich, and appendix, and I have more than my share, but dock I will pay as soon as I can get two it if you will wait, and I am going to pay You intrest on this money, ure kind dear Sir but please do not push me too fast on this money, and honest to God I'll pay you Dock.

There was also a report from the office of the County Board of Education, and I read with great interest that if the country school teacher planned his work carefully, he could keep the number of his classes down to twenty a day! I'll keep my job, thanks.

I picked up the morning paper but was called to the door. A meek-looking man asked for the doctor. I asked him to wait until the doctor returned from a call. His reply to that was, "Sorry but I don't believe I can." The young girl with him spoke in a trembling voice, "He cain't wait, Mrs. Dr., his brother stabbed him."
As they walked down the steps, I could see blood running down his legs. Later when awake in the night I thought of him and wished that I knew how he fared.

There were a few minutes left to use the typewriter, so I dashed over to the office to get it. Saw lots to do. Picked up here, and there, and dusted a bit. A patient came in who had been in an accident. He was driving a truck from Albany, New York, to Columbus, Ohio, and was pushed off the road, according to his story. He had a very bad head wound. I tried to make him comfortable during his wait for Jerry. When I asked him how far it was from Albany to Columbus, he said, "Oh, about ten cups of coffee."

Back to the house with the typewriter, I put up a card table and began to write. The table wobbled, and I struck a wrong letter. The vegetable truck arrived, and I went out to cull his stock. Back to typing. Aunt Lydia was sitting by the fire leafing through the stack of three Sunday papers which she reads on Monday. Jerry wonders if it could ease her conscience if she knew they were printed on Saturday.

The rattle of the papers dispelled the dozens of things I had been wanting to write down all morning. With quiet politeness, I offered to

help Aunt Lydia fold them. This we did, and then she began to poke
the fire, also to make several trips to the kitchen to bring one small
lump of coal at a time in a Scott paper towel. (That is one use they
do not advertise.) I typed one line. The phone rang, and it was Jerry
who had just entered the office and wanted me to send Solomon
over to get material for a temporary splint. Aunt Lydia realized that
I was trying to use the few free minutes to write, so went up to her
room.

I started again. Solomon knocked on the door, and called, "I'm
through helping Doctor, Miss, so I'll be goin' to the garden. I'd like
it much if you would come out for a minute as to see what for me to
do."

Out I went, and we decided to gather the green tomatoes (there
proved to be 12 bushels), and glad bulbs for fear of a killing frost.
Solomon asked if he could have Sunday off, although it was not his
weekend to be off. He volunteered the information that he wanted
to visit on Sunday with a man friend's woman friend. He shields me
from the facts of life.

"She has a whole heap or half-growed up children."
"Has she a husband?"
"No, Miss."
"Is he dead?"
"No, Miss."
"Divorced?"
"No, Miss."

Back to the typewriter bringing in an armload of bronze, copper, and
yellow dahlias as I came. Typed for several minutes and began to feel
a mood coming on. A siren on the bread truck dispelled it. I snatched
a dime, and went out for the staff of life, needing just that. Seeing
my kind face, and not sensing my seething condition, the bread
man rolled up one trouser leg to show me where he was bitten by a
customer's dog. He also wanted advice about his mother's stroke. I
re-entered the house musing on the complications which the domestic urge musters.

With clenched teeth, I returned to my typing thinking it might be better if I spent my time trying to perfect a model that could be attached to the hip, and used on the run.

There were three paragraphs on the bare white sheet when Jerry came bounding in to see the morning paper. More rattles. I didn't look, but I think he bathed in it. He also snapped on the radio and listened to cricket scores from South Africa via London. Was it Harriet Beecher Stowe who wrote with a baby on her lap? Oh, for one sleeping infant, and an empty quiet room. He saw a patient entering the office, and so got up, asking, "Since you aren't busy today, my love, would you press some ties for your dear husband?" I smiled an acceptance of the Honor. The muscles involved felt a trifle stiff. He dropped a hasty kiss and hurried out.

I began again, wrote about half a page, pressed a lever to make a capital letter, and hell broke loose. Nothing worked. One desperate glance at the grandfather clock told me it was time to prepare lunch. Aunt Lydia called from her room to know if I would like to see the wedding certificate of her parents. She knows I love old family letters, and papers, but I pled for a later preview.

Prepared lunch for Nancy. Jerry came, and worked on the errant typewriter, calling for various tools and articles. I found some extra milk and made Junket for Nancy's supper. Picked up tube vanilla instead of the bottle variety. Squeezed stubborn tube strenuously. In an impudent reply, it popped out one side, and all over the front of my fresh dress.

Nancy arrived, and had lunch by the fire. She enjoyed the atmosphere so much that she dallied, and had no time left to feed the puppies, but I assured her that I could do that—again. Saw her off to school. I enjoy feeding the puppies, they so obviously find life uncomplicated, and food desirable. They are fat and round like Nancy's barrel bank, but these few weeks constrain me to remark that the barrel bank is the more satisfactory possession because it has an opening in one end only.

Back to finish lunch for Lydia and Jerry. It is too early for them to
eat with Nancy at 11:30. After that, lunch for Solomon, and Pleasant,
our one-man laundry. I overheard them discussing the main theme
in Solomon's life, playing the numbers. He spends all his leisure time
working on his own scientific approach and hits just often enough
to keep him on Olympus. Last week he dreamed of his sister-in-
law, played 884, and won $9.00 on a two-cent bet. I have frequently
offered to bet with him that he will not hit, but he shakes his head
wisely, and says, "I couldn't let you do that, Miss. You'd lose money."
He mostly picks his number by the position of the hands in the com-
ic strips. For this reason, he buys a daily paper although he cannot
read.

While they talked high finance and ate a budget lunch, I stood at
the mahogany sideboard and scratched down some notes. After the
lunch series, I began again to type. Solomon called, "Miss, we had
ought to can tomatoes today."

I told him to bring them in, seeing red as I did so. Found myself
humming the childhood hymn, "Bring them in, Bring them in, Bring
them in from the fields of sin."

Away typewriter. After all, what does it matter? What I have to say
isn't meat for posterity to get its teeth into. The family's vitamins and
happiness are my paramount concern. I decided to do some rough
ironing before time to do the tomatoes, catsup this time. A knock
at the door admitted my grocer. He had his usual cup of coffee
and beamed when I paid him $13.00 on a $30.00 bill. (A lady never
mentions money, says Kathleen Morris. That lets me out, as I find it
omnipresent, and it will break out occasionally into conversation.)

When he had gone, I gathered up pencils, and notepaper, and placed
them conveniently to the right of the ironing board. Started to iron,
pressing ties before the iron got too hot, breaking speed records. I
mused to myself that the national husking contest wouldn't interest
me, but an ironing one might, and then perhaps the National Husking Champions might vie in a radio spelling match with the National

Ironing Champions. Ironing brings out the beast in me. There may be some who can sing or exercise to beautify their figures while they iron—I merely blister my hand, and my disposition.

When I began to sort the rough dry clothes, I discovered with mild dismay that Lydia had contributed to the weekly wash much long underwear, and flannelette nighties from the attic, not to be worn, but just to have them clean. If we ever build again, will there be an attic? I pressed them very sketchily feeling confident as I pressed one long leg after another (we are a long line of long limbs) that the world is growing better despite Munich.

The underwear recalled to memory the time when Nancy, not yet four, saw Aunt Lydia in her underwear, (faulty timing on Lydia's part). Nancy looked interested, and said, "Why, Aunt Lydia, you look just like the man the Good Samaritan pulled out of the gutter."

Oh, for a dull mind. I tried to shut off the thinking processes while I ironed, but instead, thoughts ran riot to the accompaniment of door, and telephone calls, and often I set the iron down to scribble a few notes. Occasionally, I looked out the window at the glorious fall colors in the garden and longed to be out close to them. On the November day, a rare armistice left the garden a blaze of glory. There were still quantities of roses, marigolds, snapdragons, calendulas, pinks, pansies, stocks, nasturtiums, chrysanthemums, violas, zinnias. To one who loves a garden Fall is as full of beauty and promise as Spring, but this day I thought a warmer gleam would light my eye if I could see a good pile of strawy manure ready to tuck the borders to sleep. The first wish if my fairy godmother finds me by the fire some evening (fat chance) will be for manure and lots of it. Whenever I want it. As it is now, I scan the horizon in daylight trips and sniff the air at night, hoping to discover an orphan pile that craves adoption.

Ironing the bath towels reminded me of the New England flood and that Nancy had a report to prepare on it. I stopped long enough to locate current papers and magazines in which she could find reports of the storm. Ironed for a half-hour, put the tomatoes to simmer, then returned to my long-suffering typewriter. With mixed emotions, I discovered that since Jerry had repaired it, none of the keys on the right half of the keyboard would return to position after being pressed. For a short time, I pulled each back by hand. Aunt Lydia called down to ask if pä and mä or pă and mă was the more acceptable pronunciation. I wanted to suggest pappy, but I was brought up too well, if wisely. Jerry breezed in from the office saying, "Will you make some tea if I put on the water?" He was preparing to lance an infection on the hand of a neighbor who had been suffering for several days and wanted an anesthetic. He drafted me in to help. The operation was a simple one, but I stayed on for a while to wash dishes which had accumulated because of her illness. Brought home her little five-year-old who is a great favorite of this family. I promised to send food in for their dinner.

When we opened our front door, we were met with a burning odor. The tea kettle had been set on the stove in fluid-less condition. Repaired the damage and served tea which refreshed the family. It does not have seven delicious flavors, but it does restore the desire to live along about 4:30 P.M.

Jerry attacked the typewriter with renewed vigor and with emphatic expletives said that we must have a new one at once. I resolved to myself that I'd rather have something substantial to fill my maid's uniforms.

Typewriter fixed—for the third time, I inserted the sheets and tried to level the line. Slipped off one shoe and began with vim. Did not feel great calm or concentration. Answering the doorbell brought me face to face with the Fuller Brush man which made me feel giddy as I knew no one would believe that. After I had eased him off the porch, without even waiting for a gift brush, I decided to relax for a few minutes, not because I needed it, but just because they say one should. I locked the front door, stretched out on the floor in front of the fire, put *The Seven Pillars of Wisdom* under the bad place in my back, and closed my eyes. Was deliciously semi-conscious when the stirring roll of a drum startled me. Gritting my teeth, I went out to watch the town's chief civic interest—the high school band—marching with great gusto out our street to test their skill and my nerves. There are children in our community without shoes but $1500 for new band uniforms is the *dernier cri*. (They got them.)

Back to what I had once thought was my avocation. Well started, when Nancy came in from school with a friend whom she wished to keep for dinner. I cordially insisted that she stay, and she took our little neighbor and went out to play with the puppies. For some few minutes, I typed in peace. Lydia offered to fry the ham for dinner, and I acquiesced. It wasn't long before I realized that the house was full of smoke, but my chapter was finished, and I went out to round off dinner, turning on the electric fan to rid the kitchen of smoke.

Dinner for six. Candlelight. Peace.

Jerry hurried with his dessert and asked me to go with him to make a call. I took my coffee and the evening paper. He stopped by the fence in front of a dooryard a short distance from town. Instead of reading I helped put 152 turkeys to bed on high wooden supports. They needed much encouragement, and I learned that they sleep there winter and summer. Why they don't freeze, I wouldn't know. They kept a suspicious eye on me to see if I had Thanksgiving intentions. How could they know that our holiday meats are usually on the bill? How they chattered at the interference. It sounded like the conversation of one I know. She asks continuous questions without ever waiting for an answer so if you insist on taking part, you have a form of conversational duet in constantly increasing crescendo. The man of the house was coming up over the hill from a spring, carrying two large buckets of water. Suddenly an upstairs window was thrown up and an angry voice shouted, "Dave, you put them buckets down. Quit doin' that female's work and maybe she won't be so lovin' to you."

The voice belonged to a jealous mother who had managed to keep a son and daughter unmarried for many years. When the son, past 40, finally eluded her and brought home a young wife, the mother became so angry that she moved upstairs, and there she stays, having no traffic with the first-floor occupants. When rural electrification came to them, she further enjoyed her martyrdom by refusing to have electricity in the upstairs. She sets oil lamps in her windows to show the public that she must use oil while the unappreciative downstairs has electricity. This condition has been going on for ten years and seems satisfactory to all.

A young son in the family came out as I got back in the car and read the evening paper. I was entranced with his scarlet hair, his freckles, and his lack of inhibitions. He did most of the talking. "Did you go to church yesterday? Boy, I did but they only got two cents out of me. I saved this (holding three pennies on his grimy palm). Boy, we had a choir I can tell you, five kids and one man. Boy, did we hop to it on 'The Old Rugged Cross.'"

We hurried home to office hours, and I went in to help Solomon finish the dishes. He neglects the last few swoops that bring final order out of confusion. Sometimes in the night when Jerry is OB-ing, I remember such insignificant details as the extremely long and sharp knife he carries. But I'd rather take chances on stabbing than do the dishes all the time, so I push disturbing thoughts into the background.

Gently I guided Nancy's storm report and checked to see if her problems were correct. She and I did exercises for her arches and practiced some dance steps. I saw that her teeth bands were clean, and the bath started. While she bathed, I freshened up again, then tucked her in and hurried down to dampen clothes and do a little more ironing. Still at it when Jerry came in. He hates to see me iron, even if I conceal it from the public. He offered me a bone disguised as the local movie with *The Texans*. I remembered a dim and distant resolve to be a helpmate and wondered if I would have enough strength to let Nancy form her own ideas on religion and companionship in marriage.

As we sat in the unventilated movie house, I watched a herd of some sort thundering over the brow of a hill. I've seen the same scene innumerable times, but for all I know, this one may have been the rear ends of the elephants in Babar. Ask me nothing more. I sat unconscious with one shoe loose. I roused once during the blood-curdling serial, when I thought the black hooded Demon had seized my foot. It was only a little boy who was searching for two pennies. He finally gave up and fell asleep. The young mother had three other children with her—all asleep. Then she left, she carried one, dragged one, of the two others, one wept loudly for his lost fortune.

I sensed that Jerry was about to leave. The accommodating owner of the movie house came and offered to run the first part of the evening's program over for us, as he often does, but I thanked him warmly and refused as gently as I could and still be firm. The lights came on, and we found two grimy pennies and gave them to the owner of the house for the little boy if he returned.

As we came out, there was a patient waiting to ask about some medicine. Also, several friends wanting to play bridge. Good host that he is, Jerry said, "Sure, come on out." I thought of three better words but added support to Jerry's invitation. Home-we-came, and began to play bridge in catsup-laden air. There were, fortunately, five, so I excused myself and went out to bottle the catsup and make sandwiches and coffee. Jerry had only played for a few hands when someone came for him and needed him right away. I became an unwilling fourth and seemed to get all the cards in the deck. Most of us are individually at our best under pressure and with our backs to the wall but there are times when I'd rather have mine on a bed. When Jerry came in, he said to me privately, "Hell, that was once when I was really needed. The patient's rupture had broken through the skin and her insides were laying in the great out-of-doors."

The guests departed about 1 A.M. and with the aid of the balusters, I made it upstairs. I must remember to have a sturdy stair rail if we build again. I was still conscious and wondered if *Good Housekeeping* would like to make me a workable schedule. I also thought that I could name one of the major causes of social unrest.

The only extra-curricular things I could recall for the day were:

> Sorted the mail twice.
> Put away the grocery order.
> Gathered fresh roses.
> Hasty glance through *Harper's Bazaar.*
> Inspected neighbor's new washer.
> Cleaned the bread box.
> Dusted the house.
> Fed the puppies and Hitty three times.
> Sewed down one rose on the quilt and one button on Jerry's vest.
> Hooked about a five-foot strip into the rug.
> Rushed out when Jean fell.
> Gathered in the clothes.
> Answered door and telephone s-teen times, nicely too!
> Read one story in *Harper's,* propped on ironing board.
> Took dinner to the neighbor.
> Dashed to the office five times.

I was nearly asleep when the phone rang. Jerry answered and I heard him say, "Then you should take her on into the hospital and I'll come right down. I'll make all the arrangements." I heard him call the hospital to reserve a room but did not hear him leave. It is irrelevant that I dreamed I was "Queen of a Green Tomato Festival."

Monday was not an unusual day. They are all like that. Sometimes the pace gets to be a little too much, and I break out in a light touch of insomnia. A professional friend suggested that it might be my arches.

[*Note: A single woman who slept with a piece of wedding cake under her pillow was thought to dream of her future husband. In this case the tradition has been adapted a bit to draw a name instead of dreaming.]

The Help
—Solomon—

[This chapter in two parts, could be titled the "Two Sides of Marriage, or Venus and Mars." Two of her helpers give their thoughts on marriage: one a man, Solomon, and the other, a woman, Susie. This chapter is a touch risqué at times, but is presented in Cornelia's general approach to life, with honest directness and pointed wit. Her ear for dialect and dialogue is gifted.]

Those help-less, self-righteous spells of self-abnegation do not occur often, and they dwindle in intensity. One day the realization will overtake me that I seem to have no more cash than when I had a substantial substitute in the kitchen. Next, I hire a promising candidate, and we are off with high hopes. I ease my conscience regarding finances by thinking of all that I learn from the help, one of whom impressed upon me that whooping cough could be cured by cutting off some of the victim's hair, mixing it with butter, spreading it on bread, and feeding it to the dog.

Without Solomon, I'd surely never know to pound rusty nails in trees to prevent fruit from dropping. Or that bean pods, spread in garden paths, produce heavy crops. I have learned that if my left eye jumps, I'm about to become very angry, if the right one performs, I'll soon be very glad. If a picture falls and doesn't break, someone in the family will die. Anyone who is hit with a broom will soon go to jail.

I'm sure that without his sage advice I would not know the proper way to conduct myself when about to be stabbed. "When a man tries to shoot or stab you, Miss, don't run, jest walk right towards him or elsen stand still. He won't shoot less'n he sees you is scared. Stay with the right people, Miss. Down South when a colored man gets in cou't (court) the Mr. Sheriff says, 'What kinda peoples does this here prisoner get hisself seen wif, the good colored or the low colored?' If they say the good colored, he doan go to the jailhouse. Missy, we needs to be careful of the people we is wif."

He told me, too, how to handle the drouth question. "Why doan you pray, Miss? Down in Georgia when they needs rain they jest prays. Why I saw the time when everything was like to blow away in dust. They all prayed loud end afore they lef the church, a cloud busted."

Solomon offered Jerry a sure cure for rheumatism and can't understand why he doesn't use it for his patients. When he was a young man, he had rheumatism so badly that he couldn't walk for a year. The woman-he-should-have-married went to the swamps and gathered barefoot (Bearfoot?) roots. She simmered half of them in a cup of lard. She divided a quart of whiskey, and added barefoot root to one portion, then she made him sip the latter while rubbing the affected parts with the lard and root concoction. A pint of plain whiskey followed. It cured him completely, and he hasn't had a touch of it for 40 years, he says.

I am told we don't need new-fangled chemists if we are careful not to begin new tasks on Friday, and we watch the Almanac signs. Gardening advice is endless. If I have the grass cut when the almanac says the sign is in the heart, it will die. If I do not want a tree to sprout, I must cut it when the sign is in the heart. The roots will then die, and soon I'll be able to shake the dead stem. I must plant grasses in the dark of the moon, or they will not endure dry spells. If I plant beans when the sign is in the arms, they will bear luxurant, but if I defy the fates when the sign is in the feet, they will not climb—just lay flat on the ground, hiding their faces in shame for my ignorance. If the sign is in the flower when the poor little beans are covered up to await their destiny, they will all go to vines and flowers. When my potatoes are covered with warts and knots, it is because I ordered their internment when the sign was in the toes. Pumpkins must not be planted when the sign is in the flower. The time for melon seed is when the sign is in the bowels. I wonder if there is any significance that melons give me indigestion.

I understand Methuselah better since Solomon came, whose age I estimate to be approximately 200 judging from the years he says he spent at dozens of occupations. He claims to be 65. He spent several periods of his life working for different families of the Socialist Register. He owned 3 or 4 farms, so spent years farming. He was a Ginner in a cotton mill for 4 years and operated a syrup mill for 7. For a long time, he was the Parter (parted those fightin') at a gin house. He carried two guns and could shoot with both at the same time. He ran a grist mill for 5 years, and after that had a hog partnership with a white man. For another long period, he agented, and made quite a bit extra besides his $200 yearly salary. He bought stolen bales of cotton for $15 and sold them for $50. He trafficked in bootleg whiskey, persimmons, backbones of fifty hogs yearly, and parched peanuts. The whiskey was kept in jugs fastened to an old log that was submerged in a pond. White people used to come to his place and eat so many peanuts that they would wade in hulls up to their knees.

Ten years he spent as political go-between for the white people and his own race, getting votes for the High Sheriff. This paid good dividends as he never had trouble with The Law. For 5 years he was well paid by owners of a still to sit high in a tree watching for the law, anti-dating the flagpole sitters. He was a Hider-of-Slot-Machines for an indefinite period, also a writer of numbers. In his fav-or-ite southern city, he held the important position of Hauler of Post-es for the city. Long experience at overseeing the planting of thousands of acres of pecans augmented his gardening lore. He's did everything, but actoring, and he thinks he could have done that.

When he came north he worked in restaurants, carpentered, was a porter in stores, did odd jobs of all sorts, worked in a mill for years and years, and dabbled in all available governmental alphabetical projects. He sighs over Friday tasks because, "It's Hangin Day." He has several children by a wife with whom he lived for 30 years. "Some

Wimin just shouldn't be married that long, Miss. The two wurst things there is, is smokin' chimneys, and quarrelsome wives. They can't be fixed. The best thing to do with both is to get yo'self a new one. Mine didn't drink whiskey or rub snuft, but I told her when the time come that she believed a $2.50 alarm clock about when I got in instead of the time I said, it was quittin' time. She didn't understood men, Miss. Men and dogs has got business out of doors. It's men's porography. He is slightly deaf which has definite advantages on many occasions.

I have been impressed not to take words too literally. Solomon was discussing truthfulness with me, "People means to be honest, mostly. My uncle's ex-wife's sister Hallie, she says she's 37." And when I asked her true age, Solomon replied, "She means to tell the truf, Miss. She might be 37 not counting all the years she went around barefoot."

He told me about Brother Corry who, alas, trusted the spoken word. During a heated revival, the congregation shouted and stamped until the red-hot stove fell down. The preacher shouted, "Pick it up, my brethren! We're in the Lord's house, so it won't burn you. Pick it up fast. "Brother Corry did as he was bade, then yelled, 'Like Hell, it won't, Brother!'"

And then there was Sister Hawkins who came in very late to church one snowy night and walked over to the old round stove. As a rebuke, the minister said, "Sister Hawkins will now pray the closing prayer." "Pray yo-self," she shouted, "You'a ought to know better than to ast a body who has walked three miles and hasn't had time to take off her boots and fascinator."

He prayed.

When on rare occasions I find that I am sympathizing with myself as a housekeeper, parent, secretary, companion, nurse, I think of an older couple, Hazel and Ralph, who worked for us, and immediately rejoice at my personal good fortune. She had a harassed expression.

He came in suspiciously quiet, and uncertain of footing after week-
ends off. Pleasant called him our retired tramp. The wife had come
from a superior family, had married against family consent, and had
spent a life of misery. She told me with whipped calm about the
night her twin girls, aged four years, both died of Black Diphtheria.
She was entirely alone. The town was having such a scourge that
neighbors were afraid to come in, and the undertakers would not
embalm or clothe the dead bodies. She held them in her arms until
each had died, then dressed them, and wrapped each in a clean sheet,
and handed them to the undertaker who would not enter the house.
In speaking of it she said, "I knew if I lived through that night, I'd
never need anyone. I had experienced the worst, nothing could ever
hurt me again."

THE HELP
—Susie—

Susie is a precious jewel that I would not trade for anyone I know
of. She would live with me all the time, (I'm her baby and I love it)
but occasionally her conscience gets the better of her and she goes
home to sew up the children or to plant the corn—she calls it serving Mammon.

I often wish I could safely express myself as graphically as she does.
On the glorious spring morning when I found the first tulips and
daffodils bursting from the ground, Susie stood in the middle of
the yard, waving her arms joyously. I asked, "What are you doing,
Susie?"
Susie replied, "Just bein' thankful I'm not in the penitentiary."
"But you never were."
"No, but if I was, I couldn't enjoy being here out of doors." I wasn't
sure that the dishes and the ironing weren't associated with the peni-
tentiary thought.
She called to Howard that he shouldn't lie on the ground, "You'll
ketch cold in your hips."

I examined the full buds on the fruit trees and remarked that I did hope they wouldn't freeze. Susie assured me, "They won't. Two years ago, God gave us plenty and we wasted it. Last year, He held out on us and gave us nothing. This year, He will try us again. There won't be any freeze." (There wasn't.)

Susie is only semi-superstitious. Sometime after she was given the clothes of a man who had killed himself, she got out a pair of shoes to wear in the garden. She set them on the table and addressed them and their former owner, "Now, Joseph, I'm goin' to leave these here for 15 minutes. If you want them, take them now and if not, I start wearing them."

She is married to a meek little man about half her size, who is definitely not the attraction at home. She discusses her personal problems with great relish and abandon while we work together enjoying household tasks of long duration. In a different day and time, she could be another Cornelia Otis Skinner [humorist for the *New Yorker* magazine] for the art of monologue is her chief delight.

As we work, she rankles along, "You wait to see him. How did I know he would look like Pharaoh's horse, and I like Adam's ox? What I can't stand is people who can eat us all away from the table and still look like their bones was too loose. All most men want is a little love and a little coffee, and they don't care where they get either one. But I shouldn't blame him—he just ain't situated for the job." She shifted from sandwiches to salad with no break in the stream of her words or consciousness.

"Can I help it if I don't love him? Or if I've been in love with someone else all my life? My mother wouldn't let me marry the man I wanted to marry, and she won't let me get a divorce. And she's had FIVE husbands!" she jabbed so viciously with the paring knife that she cut her hand. It did not interrupt the flow of words. "The Lord in his goodness removed her mistakes and had given her four new chances. She couldn't begrudge me two, cat-sneeze-it!"

I was inclined to agree but hurried with our task and let her monopolize the conversation. Jerry asked her one day how her husband was, and she jovially replied, "Lawsy, Doctor, you know he ain't serviced me for ten years."

Her eighth child was then seven, metamorphosed on Sundays into an angel in the Junior Choir by the mere addition of a choir cape, which in its previous state was a well-worn pillow slip.

Her monologues and discourses on marriage are priceless and uninhibited. I wish I could remember them all verbatim. Her sense of humor is, mostly, but not always, on sex. Last housecleaning time she, with several others, was washing the walls and ceilings. The conversation was largely Susie's.

"Ladies, there's nothin' that helps massage ceilings better than analyzin' marriage. I don't mean to be personal, Maggie, but have you got happiness?" She did not wait for an answer. "All I want is just what the good Lord intended all his children to have—a man whose mind isn't always on cows and horses. Did you ever try to drive a team of horses and one goes up and one back? (gestures). That's marriage."

"Your husband had ought to be your sweetheart, but is he? Not mine. How many Mr. Husbands go and jump in the frog pond, like Maria's did, just because we has a sweetheart? But I don't know any better place for most husbands than frog ponds, do you, Ladies?"
"One husband is enough—too much salt spoils the soup—but we do need one."

"When does a wife get her praise? In her casket with wife number two lookin' on! When she's alive, if he fails, it's her fault; if he makes it go, it's his'n. But don't never wish they was dead because they always come home those nights spryer than ever, and boy do they like to strut in late after supper is over and the dishes and babies put to bed, and you got your shoes off a-restin' your poor tired feet. That, my friends, is where the love stuff comes in."

"You turn in and cook supper again, and wash the dishes again, while he props his feet up on the stove again, and you hope he burns them."

"The greatest trouble with men is that they develops a cessation of courtin'. They all say, "I feeds you and I clothes you. What more do you want! Do I have to work all day and kiss you all night? I'm willin' to pay my fare after I ketch the streetcar, but I won't keep chasin' it.

"I've learned a lot from livin' with that man. I used to haul coal, plow the fields, and have babies all the same day, without one kind word from one week to the next. I'd even get down on my knees and beg him to be as nice to me as he was to the dog. When I had my first baby, he refused to go for help until I had cooked his breakfast so I would pour buckwheat batter on the griddle, lie down on the floor until a pain had passed, get up to turn the pancake, ditto, ditto, until his stomach was nigh as full as mine.

"I took such good care of him when he was sick that he thought he was going to graduate from the hospital to my affections. When he came home, I made him comfortable and said goodnight, but I had to turn my head so he wouldn't see me laughin'. He sat there just like a cat that sees the cream jug out of reach." *

"When I git old, I hope I won't be an old fool. All I want is chickens, a cat, a dog, a pig and one small room with a single bed. If I feel the urge comin' on, I'm goin' to pretend I'm crazy so they'll take me away. I don't know about wimin, but they always say there is danger as long as a man can carry a bushel of oats. You know old Deacon Brown, he's 92. Someone asked him how old you had to be to lose your interest in wimin and he squeaked, 'You'll have to ast an older man'n me.' Ugh, he wouldn't be appetizin' to me, would he to you, Maggie? Keep on working, Ladies, you don't have to stop work gist to talk."

Susie is much interested in spasmodic dieting, as aren't we all? She is not interested in the fit of her clothes, but she doesn't want the Lord to be ashamed of one of the things he created, and she doesn't want the undertaker to see her in her present shape. I gave her a series of exercises to take morning and night for 15 minutes at a time. The next morning, I asked her how she got along. She rolled her eyes and heaved, "Honey, 15 minutes of that would kill the horse I bought for 15 cents." (A neighbor was hired to kill and bury an old horse. Susie's entire worldly wealth was 15 cents which she offered him for the horse. He took it and his inertia and departed, leaving her to hold up the horse.) "I tried them for 5 minutes, praying all the time for strength, then I got down on my knees and prayed harder, 'Oh, Lord, let them sleep late this morning. Give me jest a half hour to rest these poor old kinks and I'll try'em again tonight but I'm not sure it's worth it, Lord!'"

A favorite expression of hers is, "I don't eat much. I jest seem to git fat on the food I think about, but don't ever offer me applesauce, that's all he cooked when I was in bed with the babies." Looking me over quizzically, she remarked, "Some women was built for pleasure and some for babies. I guess I was made for the family business." Her surmise was evident, but I chose to appear dense.

To Susie, Jerry is tops. He occupies a pedestal higher than any the rest of us perch on. When she was ill she told me, "He says I'll get better, so I'm as good as well. When he says I've got to die, I'm goin' to close my eyes and know my time's come with no foolishness."

When her sister lost a baby, it bothered Susie that her doctor was not the one in charge. She tried to comfort her sister, "We did what we could. After all, we are only Mary and Martha. If Jesus (Jerry) had been here, Lazarus would not have died."

The Bible furnishes her with much of the material for her expressive vocabulary. Watching a severe sleet storm, she observed, "Somebody'll be seein' Jesus tonight."

She has a great interest in chicken raising and on a recent trip she referred to tourist cabins with a knowing twinkle as 'Brooder Houses.' Susie thinks temptations should be avoided whenever possible. It is a premise of her philosophy that one should not trust himself too far. She urged me to keep money out of sight from the front door. "Don't leave money on your desk, Miss Cornelia. David didn't have an evil thought in his head until he looked out the window and saw that woman takin' a bath on the back porch." I am endeavoring to keep our porches above reproach.

Hired girls? Home-made-to-order gardeners? I wouldn't do without them. They enjoy life so thoroughly that they enrich our own life enjoyment.

Not Just Case Histories

[While researching Dr. Jerry and Cornelia Thompson, everyone I spoke to said he was a wonderful doctor. Many remember going to him as a child, and none had anything but warm and fond memories.]

A doctor's wife soon learns to prepare for long waits in the car, not all of which can be anticipated. I keep a supply of magazines, books, and seed catalogues near the front door so that I can refuel without stopping. I also carry sewing and knitting as standard equipment. An eleven-year-old is not well geared to indefinite waiting so even Nancy rushes to find puzzles, dolls, *Child Life*, or a book.

My long waits when Jerry is making calls present a large screen with constantly changing scenes. I do not always read. Today is Sunday. The sun is defying the approach of Winter, but it is a deceptive siren for I shivered when I first went out. I had planned to read while he made the call but in a vacant field, where the barren weed stalks waved farewell to summer as she drew her garments closer and fled over a far hill, an old lady stood with her cow. She was clad in somber black. Heavy boots peeped from beneath a shabby hem. An old red knit cap of nondescript design concealed all but a few wisps of discouraged gray hair. She was near enough that I saw deep wrinkles, like longitudinal valleys, running from brow to chin through the clay borders of her cheeks. Time and again she jerked on a dirty rope that was knotted around the horns, trying to draw attention to choicer salad for the feast.

The backdrop was a dilapidated wooden paling fence, gray from weathering and no paint. Just beyond was a hay mound topped with a square of once-white oilcloth. I left the car and the book I had planned to read and approached to see if my vision was reality. She smiled and I marveled at the expression. There was friendliness and pleasure, more too—a kindliness that was a composite of her youthful dreams, her work in the soil, the children and animals she had tended. I smiled too. Instead of telling her that I was remembering moon shadows through an old church window, I said, "A fine place for your cow."

"Nice place," she smiled.

"Doesn't it tire you to lead her?"

"No, this Sunday. I give Anna change. I like. She like."

"I like too," I said as I patted Anna.

She was not a golden yellow cow with a heavy udder, nor yet one of sharp black and white contrasts. She was like human animals who have no perceptible coloring—neutral—with eyes that may once have been blue, but they were expressionless black—solid blotches like ink dropped on a blotter.

Poor Anna? Not at all. Anna gives her mistress pleasure, who must sometimes long for the hills of her homeland. Anna helped me too. I shall try to be more charitable toward those who like to be led by a rope around their horns—because of a sunny fall Sunday when I met Anna.

Books I have read on long waits have strange associations for me, viz:

> *Bulwark of the Republic*...Pus tubes.
> *The Flowering of New England*...Twins.
> *An American Doctor's Odyssey*...Heart Attack.
> *Inside Asia*...Gall Stones.
> *Madam Curie*...Cancer
> *Gone With the Wind*...Convulsions.

But whatever the association, they are blessed companions and have probably prevented a divorce in the family. Whether the ever-present books on Obstetrics, Urology, Pediatrics, and General Medicine are good reading for the younger generation of our family remains to be seen. If I'd seen one as a child, I'd have read it in the haymow. Nancy reads them in the living room, occasionally asking calmly, "Is this true?"

Medical magazines of a dozen different brands complicate house-keeping in every room in our house. They increase and overflow like the offspring in Pigs is Pigs. It is difficult for me to be ruthless with such vast knowledge. I decide we need the use of some of the tables and chairs and start to gather them up only to see on one unassuming cover, such overwhelming subjects as:
   Strongyloidiasis
   Fatal Granulocytopenia (no wonder)
   Chronic Adhesive Spinal Arachnoiditis

Respect and awe, slightly seasoned with mirth, surge over me, but I steel myself, sandwich a few between *TIME* and *Good Housekeeping* and give them to the Salvation Army to worry about. For awhile I sent copies of various magazines to the local branch of the Carnegie Library, but when there were never any calls for them, I decided that their value as waste paper to the Salvation Army outweighed that as shelf filler to the library.

I browse through many medical articles and frequently look at the impressive case histories. They look and sound like casualty lists:

   Case XXX11,
   Male,
   White,
   Age 57,
   Entered 4/10/38 etc.

It sounds like the reports on the "Farm and Home" hour or the activities of the Stock Exchange.

It is impossible to assume the detached attitude toward patients that many times we wish we had.

I do not see number X11,
male child,
12 years old

When I watch Billy riding his bicycle or roller skating. Rather, I remember that he lay completely pulseless on the operating table and caused breathless moments to several M.D.'s who tried every known method of resuscitation before he rallied. I am glad his parents did not know the fright, and I feel a warm inner glow that he is now scurrying people off the sidewalk as he skates or rides.

I wish the enormous energies of young Tobey could be diverted and directed. At a very undernourished four years of age, he sat on the operating table with a broken arm and a bleeding head and defied an over-nourished professional man in language most astounding: "I betcha by gawd you better let my head alone. I betcha by gawd you better not touch my arm, you sumabitz or I'll sock you one between the eyes." He is better now, I saw him able to sock one—one day last week. His language was a contrast to that of a young nephew of mine who while visiting us, also at the age of four, wished to express anger in vile terms to relieve a feeling of great annoyance toward his sister. He sputtered with venom, "Why, you—you, you're nothing but your mother's child!"

Sophia is not just a foreign patient with too many children, but is a woman of heroic courage in facing poverty, disaster, or suffering. She has managed through the depression to keep her large family clothed and fed without aid from any of the charities and with no complaints. She suffered for weeks with badly congested breasts, and when Jerry scolded her for not coming to him sooner, she replied, "But Doctor, no work, no moneys. Nothing to pay Doctor." And to think of all the thankless work he does for nothing.

Ruth, aged seven, has recovered from a serious case of pneumonia, but in having it she provided the means for her parents to have the time of their lives. They live on an inaccessible farm with her parents. The purse strings are pulled tight by the older generation, where they're not loosed to treat for "foolishness." The young parents had never had a honeymoon, been away from home, or spent any money for pleasure, so in spite of the worry, they loved every minute of the child's illness in the hospital. They ate in restaurants and went to several movies. He bought her a box of candy! Jerry was sorely tempted to hospitalize Ruth longer than necessary. He was not merely the medical mentor but was indirectly the means of providing the parents with a new horizon they had only dimly suspected.

Our contact with the Thomas Browns is more than a complicated case history, it is an entire chapter in our lives. It began before our marriage. I was driving in the country one day without Jerry. I saw two elderly people gathering cherries. She, a tiny female gnome, was up at the top of an unsteady ladder. He, a lumbering giant, sat on the lowest round. I stopped to buy some cherries. As I was leaving I told them that I was interested in buying old furniture and thought perhaps they could direct me to some. They looked at each other significantly, but said they knew of none. Several days later I returned the pail and Emmy invited me in. She began showing me furniture she wanted me to buy, and before I left that day I had acquired a beautiful bed, two Windsor rockers, and a mahogany chest. They both told me that they did not need to sell the pieces, but they wanted me to have them because they were growing old, and what relatives they had were eagerly waiting to grab their things, so they decided to dispose of them as they pleased.

A short time after that, Tom was driving sheep along the highway when a hit-and-run driver knocked him down, leaving him with a compound leg fracture. Emmy weighs about eighty pounds. How she managed to care for him, shovel snow, tend fires, and look after the run-down farm was a constant marvel to me. When he could get around again, he was very lame, so they decided they must leave the farm.

One day when I called, they told me they had decided to dispose of all their possessions and enter a home for the aged located in another state. I discovered that they knew the place only by hearsay, so persuaded them to so on an inspection tour before making such a momentous change. They came home completely disillusioned, and we helped them pack up to leave the farm and move to a neighboring small town.

We bought more furniture, a settee with a lady's chair to match, a finger-roll armchair with six straight chairs. She gave me two beautiful sewed-on quilts, some good old glass, and wanted to give me her wedding cape, which I refused. Nancy received her plain gold ring, as no amount of persuasion could make her keep it. The relations again."

They never went anywhere so it was a gala occasion when we persuaded them to come to the fair. They stayed overnight, slept in their own bed, saw all their furniture restored, and went with us to the evening show at the fair. It was the equivalent of a European trip to anyone else.

Not long ago, Tom died a peaceful death from a malignant growth in his throat. He talked about approaching death as if he were about to go on a visit. I heard him say to Jerry, "I've lived a long time and I'm not going to start worrying now. I'll just breathe as long as I can and when its too hard, I'll go on my way."

His only worry was Emmy, whose decisions he had made for forty years. I try to see her often and remember her at various holidays. One day recently I was ironing, musing over the idea that I was surely not intended for such, with long fingers that encircle the iron handle nearly twice. Jerry came in and asked me to go to the next town with him so I could call on Emmy while he saw another patient.

I had ironed enough to ease my conscience and reduce the pile. If I persist more than two hours straight, my faith in a planned universe totters, so out we went. I called to see Emmy. She had an elderly caller. I soon realized he did not hear me. He came closer and said, "I don't hear very well. I don't see very good either, but otherwise, I feel fine. I just hitch-hiked up four miles to prayer meeting this evening. How old do you think I am?"

"Oh, about seventy," I shouted.

"No, siree. I'm eighty-eight. There are eleven people past eighty in this little town. Must be a healthy place, we are all as spry as crickets. At home I left Rachel, ninety-three, Ann, eighty-six, Samuel, eighty-four, and there's me, eighty-eight. Ann did a big wash today, on the board too. And then went out to the garden to gather green tomatoes and pepper for pickle. I bet Rachel has got more put up than anybody in this whole countryside. (If he hadn't been so hard of hearing, I'd have argued that point.)

"Yes, siree, we do all the farm work. The only trouble is, I can't drive the car. When I was eighty-three, I drove home from town one day and I couldn't tell which side of the road I was on, so I drove in the barn, patted Henry on the nose, walked in the house and told them all, 'I'll never drive again.'"

I tried to tell him I was sorry about Henry, but he interrupted me, "Oh, shucks, I don't mind a bit. I can walk all day, not bad at eighty-eight. Emmy ain't no spring chicken either, are you Emmy?" Emmy blushed and said, "I ain't tellin'."

Her caller teased, "Now, Emmy, don't you remember Betty S. who wouldn't tell how old she was, always said, 'When you see it on my tombstone, you'll know,' and she died and nobody ever gave her a tombstone!"

But Emmy still wasn't tellin', so he left to make other calls before prayer meeting and Emmy carried on. "That's true about Betty. I'm tryin' now to borry some money to buy Tom a tombstone. He said to me before he died, 'Emmy if you don't get you and me a tombstone and mark it, nobody will'. So, I gotta. And he wanted me to leave our property to the church, so I want to borry some more so I can get it fit to leave."

I'm not half as old as Ann, but I came home and finished the ironing in record time—and liked it.

Dinner was interrupted one evening by Johnny's Mother. She had Johnny in the car and both were too frightened to talk coherently. He had fallen from a tree and fractured his arm. The bone of the lower arm was protruding through mangled flesh of the upper arm. Jerry thought he should be hospitalized at once. I went along. Johnny had rare courage. I stayed by his bed in the hospital. He was in such pain that he had a hard, white line around his mouth, but he shed no tears and made no complaints.

Once he said, "If I'd minded my Dad, this wouldn't have happened. He told me not to climb that apple tree." And again, "Please go tell Mom not to worry. I'll be OK." He was such a courageous lad that I felt physically ill when it later proved necessary to amputate the arm. And I still remember the smile when he spoke of his greatest treasure, "Well, I guess I can teach sister to play my new accordion."

When Jerry was called one Sunday evening to come to St. Paul's African Methodist Episcopal Church because Mary had taken a bad spell, I went along because Mary had been like one of our family. When we parked near the church, we could sense the excitement. Mary was undoubtedly the most worthy pillar of the church. That evening she had been called on to pray and soon after she began, she fell on the floor. When we arrived, they had lifted her to the front pew. One of the parishioners was half moaning, half praying "On, Lord, send the Great Physician, we need the Great Physician." Jerry noted that his coming did not change the trend of the prayer.

The minister in his black robe was chanting a spiritual and interrupting each line to say, "We all have our time to go, to each is the appointed time." The choir and the congregation sat transfixed, some in attitudes of prayer and some wide-eyed with excitement. Several of Mary's children and grandchildren were present. There was dramatic silence when Jerry pronounced her dead. As we left, I thought how Mary would have loved the drama. She had once told me about the time a baby had been born in the little church. Her death as she prayed seemed to complete the cycle.

Mary was a town institution. All her life she had been self-supporting, in spite of a good but improvident husband. When her house burned down, even though she would normally be thought old, she had it rebuilt and worked it out. She worked for Father for years and was often left in charge of the house and boys if we were away. She always refused a high wage, saying that she prospered better on a small one. One day she said to me, "Miss Cornelia, I don't think I can wash for you much longer. When I started out to wash, I said I'd wash and support my family for fifty years, then they'd have to take care of me."

"Mary!" I gasped, "Do you mean you deliberately faced a life of washing for fifty years?"
"Why, yes, Miss Cornelia, and I've waited for nearly sixty, so I think it's time they learned to take care of me." I heartily agreed and urged her to stop that instant, but she continued to wash until she broke her wrist.

She always knew village news almost before it happened and enjoyed relaying it to me. She was completely incredulous and at a loss for words when I said to her one day, "Next week, Mary, you'll have to manage without me. (She was afraid of electricity so wouldn't use the electric stove, or have an electric washer.) I'm going to Pittsburgh to have a baby."

I laughed at her surprise. At last, she retained control of the situation. "Well, I might have knowed it, I've been praying you would."
I hadn't thought to credit Mary with my good fortune but smiled and said, "Why, thank you very much indeed, Mary. I appreciate your efforts on my behalf but do let me know before you and the Lord get together again." She agreed.

Mary had scant sympathy for any weak male who succumbed to a designing woman. "Anybody knows you can't get hold of a man who puts a dime under his tongue and salt in his shoes," She told me that one child born out of wedlock was not to be criticized but a second was inexcusable. She had eight children, seven without benefit of doctors. She explained with pride, "Of course, I had one doctor the first time because it was all new to me. After that I took care of it all myself."
I felt like a sissy going to a hospital.

Each New Year's Day, or soon after, she dressed in her best and came to call bringing a brown crock filled with baked sausage. Nobody can make sausage like Mary's. We anticipated it all year.

When she died, they found $150.00 in cash in one of her petticoats. She always had greater confidence in her petticoat or stocking than she did in man-made institutions. She prospered. I had often seen her add to her savings account.

Her funeral was all she could have desired. No, Mary was not just another patient, diagnosis: cerebral hemorrhage.

When a nice young girl had a baby she would rather not have had, to me it was not just another tragic case history. She had wanted to write poetry and had brought a book of her poems, dealing with all Life's Processes, to me for criticism. They showed some promise. One subject stands out in my mind from the others:

IN DEATH

or

LINES WRITTEN ON VIEWING A FUNERAL

I remembered that the day her baby was born. If I am around when jeweled crowns are passed out in the hereafter, I intend to say, "Just pass mine on up to Margaret." I don't care for elaborate jewels, (although I like an occasional large ring which Jerry says makes me look like a prostitute) and I can't see how anyone with a sense of humor could sparkle under a tiara, but even if I did like them, I'd still pass mine to Margaret because her best crown will be too heavy for everyday wear.

Margaret is the young mother of three. Before her last one, a little boy with blonde curls, arrived, she had nearly every known complication. They culminated in a Caesarean Section with more complications. While she was still bedfast at home, a new acquaintance, who had been at the hospital at the same time with a new baby, came to call, bringing her three year old child. Margaret held the child and noticed that it seemed lame. The mother thought it had a touch of rheumatism. Margaret has not walked from that day to this and her baby is now six. She contracted infantile paralysis from the visiting child. She cared for her new baby by having its bed put on rollers. She does all her own work with what help her husband and two little girls can give. She even manages the washing and ironing sitting in a wheelchair, with useless feet stretched out straight in front of her. She irons with the board across her legs. Much of the time she is alone on the farm. They have almost no money. She makes all the children's clothes by hand, even the little boy's overalls. She tried to get into the Warm Springs Foundation, but was not accepted. She did not voice her great disappointment.

No, Margaret is not:
Case XXX11
Age 35
Diagnosis: Infantile Paralysis.

Even though this type of medical practice adds many complications to the doctor's life and to that of his family, it adds breadth to the vision, depth to the understanding, and is a marvelous aid to diagnosis.

For example, Jerry knew that a patient who was losing weight and complaining of numerous symptoms chiefly concerning her stomach was unhappy with her husband, and to soothe her resentment had become a morphine habitué. He discouraged a suggested operation on the stomach and later when the patient's love life righted itself, she had no further complaints.

Another patient had similar symptoms of lost weight, no appetite, excessive nervousness. She was advised to have a goiter removed. Jerry was opposed to the radical treatment because he knew that only a false pride kept her living with a worthless husband. But grasping at a straw, she had the thyroid operation. Her symptoms are, the same. What she needs is the amputation of the marital tie and a rest from discord.

Another case which was solved because of a knowledge of the family background was that of an adolescent boy who was such a discipline problem at school that the authorities decided to dismiss him. We heard about it and Jerry went to the school board quietly and urged them to reconsider. He tried to explain the boy's emotional inheritance. He was the last of eight children. The parents had always quarreled, and the children were divided into two camps. Both the parents were unstable. The youngest lad was torn between his loyalties, and as a release became a troublesome young citizen. At Jerry's suggestion, he was quietly made to feel a responsible member of the whole group—not of a faction as at home. It took time and intelligent handling, but he came through in spite of the bad prognosis. He had been slated for the reform school but now is a well-adjusted father of a family.

In the bosom of the family, we often speak of one of the many cases which has helped to teach us tolerance and sympathy. For years, Edgar Jones was criticized for laziness, loss of ambition, poorly concentrated effort. Jerry knew the long family history of early arteriosclerosis, hardening of the arteries, and the many early deaths from cerebral hemorrhages. The average layman was critical and unsympathetic in his judgment, or frankly ridiculed him until he developed the inevitable symptoms which mark the progress of the disease. Jerry had understood him all along.

These isolated cases alone would justify our belief that knowledge of the sociological background is essential. It also increases and holds the interest in the patients' welfare. The work of the family doctor should never be replaced by the age of Specialists. Patients are actual human beings with complex problems and backgrounds—not just case histories.

While the Village Sleeps

["Freedom is the natural right of all men." Cornelia came from a long line of Quaker families. The Quakers, or Society of Friends, bore a testimony of equality among all mankind, male and female, regardless of race. In this chapter, and elsewhere in this book, Cornelia uses dated terminology that some may find offensive today. Clearly, she would not intend it as such.]

The papers and pictures reek of case society, or shall we say cafe society reeks? After I have been in the city for a few days and have seen the shallow repetition of the nightclubs, which I enjoy in small doses, I want to bury my face in the first field of green grass. A random thought occurs to me that if the constant go-er would drop into such places the morning after, about 11 A.M. the attendance might drop off.

We could not often be a part of it if we would nor does opportunity present itself in this wholesome town atmosphere unless we go far afield. For this, there is no time. As it is, Guiseppe's Night Club in a nearby village can offer a wheezy victrola as accompaniment for two pieces of bread with a thin shaving of ham and a smeary glass of beer.

We are supposed to have Thursday and Sunday evenings to ourselves. What we should like to do is to sit by the fire or in the garden and read, but unless we leave town, we are constantly besieged by pseudo patients at door and telephone who, "Just thought I'd find you at home." When cats, rabbits, and skunks cross our light beams at night, I often say to Jerry, "Wouldn't you think anything that could stay home—would?"

Our hours for reading are the peaceful ones from 12:30 A.M. to 2:30 A.M. (After any melee). And yet, because we sit absorbed, without conversation, one relative thinks we are not happy. A real vacation is to be away for one whole night from the telephone.

Our nightlife is time and interest-consuming. Occasionally we have a mad desire for sleep but fortunately not often. Where night clubs would grow monotonous, ours is a constant shift of scenery and props, and if we crave music, we can match our moods for swing, or sweet, or lofty, or serious, by a twirl of the dial on the dash, (if it is working) as we flit about Florence Nightingale-ing and Hippo-crates-ing.

We both wish we had Pepys-ed all these years as almost any day or night presents seemingly fictional material, some dramatic, some just mildly interesting, but nearly all are incidents we should like to remember. For example, we have been held up four times with no particularly disastrous results except to our morale. For a time Jerry carried a gun, but then every shadow, fence post, tree, or tall weed was an escaped lunatic, or the man who robbed the local bank—though why he might be interested in us I wouldn't know—so we stopped being a toy arsenal and have not been alarmed since.

About 1 A.M. one summer night we were tearing down a hill out of a little town near here when a masked figure stepped into the road directly in our path. Instead of slowing down, Jerry used all available power and drove directly at the man. He jumped out of the way so quickly that he lost his balance and fell sprawling. We allowed our normally humanitarian instincts to lie dormant and dashed madly on.

Another night we were traveling a narrow dirt road so unfrequented that a grassy lane grew in the center. Coming around a sharp turn, we nearly crashed a large touring car parked directly across the road. Two figures leaped out, both armed. My heart seemed to stop beating and I nearly swallowed a ring hastily popped into my mouth. They came and peered into our faces and one remarked to the other, "Nope, Pete, this ain't him." They straightened up their car and with exaggerated politeness directed our passing on the narrow road. As we drove on watching every shadow, my mind flashed back to the first night my eldest brother Ezra and I were permitted to take the horse and buggy for a party in the country. En route home, we both went soundly to sleep, Beauty trotting along placidly with slack reins toward home and pasture while we slept. I awoke very suddenly and was startled to see a dark figure shaking Brother, "Wake up, Bud, or you'll be landin' in a ditch—You ain't who we's expectin'."

We sat very close together until we were out of sight, then Ezra climbed out the shaft and onto Beauty's back so he wouldn't go to sleep. No one could sleep with her corrugated trotting pattern. Shivering and yawning I held the reins and wondered if grown-ups were really brave and if parties were worth the dreadful feeling then present in what I supposed was the pit of my stomach. Later my knees shook when Brother offered me five cents to go with him to hold the lantern while he put away the buggy and turned the horse to pasture. Home and bed seemed heavenly secure that night. We kept our experience a deep secret lest the family think night travel to be as dangerous as we thought it was.

Once after Jerry had spent a futile and tragic two hours helping a cancer tortured patient welcome Death, he came out to his car and found that the lights refused all persuasive efforts. The grief-stricken old man tied his lantern onto the front of the car and Jerry started off, promising to send an undertaker. He soon found the going too dangerous with the poor visibility so pulled over to sleep until daylight. He woke to find his lantern extinguished, a gun poking him in the ribs, and a nasal whine ordering from the security of a bandage, "Hand it over, Buddy."

A wallet containing $462.00 (those were the days—he hasn't had that much since!) passed from one hand to the other as Jerry said, "With the greatest of pleasure, but will you kindly remove that gun? There's something about it that I don't like." The man disappeared, Jerry re-lighted his lantern and meandered into town, completely awake. Late the next morning, he entered his office which was not locked.

On his desk, he saw a small box and this letter:

> Gosh, Dock I didn't know that was you. Jeff says you stayed with
> his missus until she died and that he put a lantern on your car.
> Gosh, I'm sorry. All I wanted was enough to buy some vittles and
> some shoes for the kids to wear to school, but I can't take your
> money, Dock. I was kinda desperate but I'm ashamed so won't
> sign my name. Dock, once you bought some special medicine for
> one of my kids when I couldn't.

Jerry brought me the note and the box at noon as a surprise, saying,
"Just so much velvet, my love. Put it in the blow-out fund. Oh, yes,
and let's remember the Waite family anonymously if the Christmas
budget can stand it."

What we believe were attempted hold-ups remain unsolved mysteries.
We were coming home after a late call one night when our lights suddenly silhouetted two figures fighting. We could see gleaming knives,
and on the road a naked body with what looked like blood smears.
We drove on debating what to do and about fifty yards ahead, a figure
rose from the ditch at the roadside and attempted to stop us. We
drove like mad and reported the incident to the nearest authorities,
but nothing came of it, nor was any mention made in the papers.

Another night in the driving rain, we saw a woman standing on a
ten-foot embankment beside the highway apparently holding a baby.
She had no umbrella or hat. I called Jerry's attention to her, but he
was on an emergency call and said we would investigate on our return
trip. We discussed the possibility of a plant and decided it would be
foolish to stop as there were three other urgent calls to make. There
were strange aspects to the case. She made no effort to stop us, or
to thumb her way. In either direction she could have reached a farmhouse in several minutes.

We were gone about an hour and coming back we anxiously watched
for the spot. She was still there, an impassive figure standing in the
pouring rain. We drove on without stopping to hurry to other calls,

yet I worried so much about her plight that we retraced our route before going home. She was still there. We hurried back to town and sent an officer out, but he failed to find her. Later we talked with people in three other cars who had seen the same thing, so we had not imagined it. It seems heartless not to stop, but we are cautious since friends of ours went to the aid of a screaming girl who was struggling with two men. The girl searched their pockets while the two men kicked and beat them.

Many nights stand out as clearly etched on my mind as if they had been photographed at the time. The events are silhouetted against shadows.

During Prohibition, there were constant bootleg feuds or wars in progress between factions of different nationalities, viz., Italian vs. Spanish vs. Bohemian. A reputed 'tough guy,' currently thought responsible for several recent deaths, called by phone in the night for the doctor. He thought his baby was dying and was sure it had pneumonia. "He's awful sick, Doctor. I'll see you safe here and back if you will come."

Jerry had no desire to become involved in the feuds, but a sick child needed attention, so we started. A convoy of four cars met us at the top of the hill out of town. Two cars preceded us and two brought up the rear of the strange procession. Jerry walked some distance from the car to the house but was well escorted.

I sat alone in the car, shivering as I'm not too brave. The lights were on dim and I could see a figure weaving up the road. My reaction was to jump out and hurry to the house, but I clenched my teeth, mentally damning if I would and sat with hand on horn. When the weaver reached the car, he examined the front tires carefully, then came and tried to open the door which I was grimly holding. I pressed the horn, no response. Any other time, it would wake the dead. In desperation, I grabbed the flashlight and flashed it in his eyes. He yelled in terror, "Don't shoot, Mister, please don't shoot!" Jerry heard the commotion, rushed out, and without too much respect for age, started my companion of the shadows double-spacing up the road.

As we started home—paid (the worse the reputation, the better the pay!)—a car at a neighboring unfriendly menage pulled out hastily. About a mile up the road they turned around hurriedly and sat with bright lights streaming our way to see who we were. Evidently, we passed muster for we reached home safely. We knew that an innocent car on a previous evening had come out with two holes in the windshield.

One night returning from a movie in town with another couple about 11:30 P.M, we saw a car overturned, so backed up to see if anyone was hurt. The car rested on its top. The occupants were screaming so lustily that our first thought was that they could not be badly hurt. Just as the boys crawled through the barbed wire fence, a farmer who lived across the road, came out, stood agape for a long minute, and then with great concern shouted, "My pig pen again. That's the third time a car has crashed it." No interest in the occupants of the car. And sure enough, one of the denizens of the pig sty lay prone under the car, the others huddled in the farthest corner.

The boys succeeded in extricating the eight passengers—four adults and four children—without the help of the farmer who was consoling his pigs. The car was badly damaged, and the occupants suffered minor injuries and cuts. They were too tightly packed in to be thrown loose from the car. A passing sedan slowed up and two people came to investigate. The occupants were engaged in some local missionary work, but they would not use their back seat to carry some of the cold and frightened colored people to the office in town. Jerry left us and took them all to the office—as patients of ours—then gave them needed care and took them home.

After Jerry had returned and collected us, he found a call to hurry to the hospital. I was too tired to be inspiring company so he hurried away. Soon after I fell asleep, I was startled by a loud noise. Screams in the night have an ominous sound, especially if one is alone. I heard loud shrieks as a car slowed up in front of the house. Jerry was out, I sighed as I hurried into my dressing gown and answered a pounding on the door accompanied by the ringing of the bell, the barking of our dog, and the thumping of my pulse. A frightened man stood at the door.

"Please, Missus. Call Doc quick!"

"He isn't here. What is the trouble?"

"Well, can we bring that woman in here? She's bleedin' to death."

"I'm sorry but this isn't the right place for that. You should hurry for another doctor."

"But, Missus, we've tried everybody else."

That is a flattering and frequent theme and is the logical place to summon the good old sense of humor. A good predecessor of ours, who devoted a long life to doctoring this community's ills before good roads or cars were dreamed of, told about a dark night when he rode horseback eight miles on mud roads accompanied by an anxious husband. About six miles out the man said, "I wouldn't have bothered you, Doc, but I couldn't get Dr. A. or Dr. B,"

The resigned physician replied, "Well, I'm not surprised that you couldn't, since Dr. A has moved away and Dr. B. is in the cemetery."

"I know, Doc, that's why I got you."

"You'll just have to do something, Missus Doctor."—Loud yell.

"Where is she bleeding?"

"Arm—she fell through a window. Please look at it, lady."

I went out to the car and had difficulty seeing because of the dark night and the fact that the patient was struggling as three men held her. All five were drunk. I marveled that the car had reached our house. Back in the house, I found some clean towels, returned, and had an uncertain gentleman help me apply a tourniquet. We had just finished the unprofessional service, with the screams piercing the dark night like ragged streaks of lightning, when Jerry pulled up. He smiled at my predicament. They carried her into the office. The night air was probably responsible for my weak thought that she should not be heavy with all that air that had been expelled from her lungs. My education was considerably augmented by a constant stream of oaths unknown to me, as Jerry sewed her up. We learned that in fighting for her favors, one of the inebriated gentlemen picked up a glass kerosene lamp and hurled it at a rival.

When the well-stitched model had departed, supported by four escorts who could scarcely stand-alone, I made some coffee and sandwiches. Over the restoring brew, Jerry told me about his trip home. At 3:30 A.M. en route home, he narrowly escaped running over the figure of a man lying in the center of the street in a suburb of the city. He stopped the car and got out. A brief examination found the old man dead. Near him lay a wet paintbrush and an upset bucket of white paint. He had been painting a center line, was struck by a hit-and-run driver and killed. Jerry called the police and drove on.

As he approached the curve on a long hill, he saw a dark figure shove a blazing touring car over a steep hill and then run out of sight into the woods on the other side of the road. After twice notifying authorities, he said he was glad to see the lights of home.

We had just sighed deeply over the vicissitudes of life, practicing medicine in the country, when the doorbell pealed.
In contrast to the hysteria with which we had just dealt, a quiet orderly gentleman, haggard with worry, stood at the door. Jerry opened the screen and said, "Who's there?"
The calmest voice I have ever heard replied in a conversational tone, "It is I, Doctor. Will you come, please? Eva—is dying."
And Jerry went—like a human cannonball. Eva still lives. The quiet voice is stilled.

Country telephone lines are not all they should be, but they do have advantages, at least to people on the lines:
   a. They make a newspaper non-essential.
   b. As a means of social intercourse, the country telephone wins hands down over afternoon teas and bridge sessions.
   c. One can conveniently pretend that the line is bad—which it usually is.

To the Country Doctor, they are a major curse as he is constantly at their beck and call. I awaken more easily than Jerry, so I usually answer the phone. One particular night, when Jerry was tired from overwork, I had difficulty getting directions even though I distinctly heard an extra receiver click and a third party say, "I guess the Dixon girl's time's come, Pa."

I went along to open gates, bags, Lysol bottles, tincture of green soap, tool kits, etc. Ever since a helpful member of the audience one night poured straight Lysol on Jerry's hands and arms instead of green soap, burning him terribly, he has preferred my assistance, though I have often heard him announce to a family, "I couldn't get any other help so I brought my wife." I want to watch his face the day I shall surprise him in that remark by saying loudly, "He didn't really try."

I helped change a tire by the light of a flashlight. I read about the kind that throws its little beam hundreds of feet into the naughty world. Ours sheds a light that resembles a weak flash from a sluggish lightning bug. I opened two gates on rusty hinges. I never open a gate, even in the middle of the night, that I don't think that I'd hate to live where they were outmoded. I love them, but perhaps more by day than at 2 A.M. We climbed a veritable mountain up over ledges of rock in a cow pasture. Once at the top, Jerry got out and said, "Come on."

I could not see where we were going but followed and soon wished I was home in my little bed. We slipped and walked down the steepest hill I ever saw. I sat down twice vehemently and through no desire of my own. At the bottom of the canyon, we crossed a small stream. There wasn't a sign of a path or bridge, so we walked through, climbed a rail fence, and started up out of the cavern. Well, nigh spavined, we approached a light in a small cabin. A man met us, saying, "Gee, I'm glad you're here. I walked two miles to the nearest phone over at neighbor Browns. His line was down, and I tied it in six places and strung it along the fence before I could get the operator."

The parents of the young mother were emotionally upset but not the patient. Jerry asked the older woman to hold the kerosene lamp for him. Everything was quiet for a few minutes. I happened to turn around and saw the human lamp post weaving. In a second both she and the lamp were on the floor. Jerry grabbed the lamp and threw it out the door where it exploded. With no words I brought a lamp from the lean-to kitchen and was forced to straddle the figure on the floor to hold the light as Jerry needed it.

As I held the lamp I marveled silently that one could live in such an inaccessible place and yet become pregnant. It strengthened my belief in the Immaculate Conception.

Riding home, I remembered that as a child I used to be impressed by hearing a minister at least semi-monthly quote with dramatic intensity what he considered an apt fragment from Shakespeare. He would wait for silence and then sepulchral tones would roll, "When graveyards yawn and all Hell breathes out contagion into the World." This made me suppose for some time that nights were necessarily wicked.

We were no more than home when Jerry answered the phone and heard, "Doctor, this is Arnold Cox. I'd like you to come out to my place. I've just shot a bunch of men and I don't know how many." We hurried out and as we neared the farm were flagged down with a lantern. It was Arnold himself, "I don't know how many got away but two of them is lying up there along the pike. I got tired of having something stolen nearly every night—hams, sheep, hay, gasoline, chickens—so tonight I just stayed up and waited for them with my shotgun. I was back of the garage when I heard a car slow up. Several men got out and started to siphon gas out of my car, not twenty-five feet from where I was hidden, so I let them have it from the shotgun."

We found the men up the road. One was sitting up, the other moaning as he lay in the ditch. Jerry examined them both and said that the one seriously injured must not be moved. He seemed to have shot all over him, so Jerry went to the house to call an ambulance.

While he was gone, I talked with the young boy who lay in the ditch. He was shivering with cold and shock. (Like Franklin, when I'm warm and comfortable I have enormous sympathy for the underdog or man.) I asked a bystander for a cover and his reply was, "Let him freeze." When he saw me taking off my coat, he went into the barn and brought out an old horse blanket. The boy was pitifully young, with fair hair and freckles. He smiled when I covered him and asked for a drink. He mumbled, "Would you put your hand on my head, it's breaking open. Today's my birthday. Swell present I gave myself. Nobody's give me a present since my mother died eight years ago. My Dad's no good. I guess I'm not either."

Jerry returned. The officers came. One came over, gave the boy a kick with a heavy shoe, and said, "Get the hell up out of there."
Jerry interrupted, "Sorry, officer, but he's not to be moved until the ambulance comes."
I asked Jerry if I could slip something under the boy's head. His reply was, "Don't be too sentimental. After all, they had this coming to them."
I needed that jerk back to reality. The officer snorted for my benefit, "Great help a woman is with the law. I suppose she thinks she would make a fine Guvnor."
A search was made, and the officers found another accomplice back of the barn. They finally loaded the one into the ambulance and made the other two get in the rumble seat of the patrol car. The prisoners asked if they might get their coats but were refused with the gruff words, "Where you're goin' you won't need no coats."
They drove off into the cold night with no protection from the weather for the handcuffed prisoners.
It was my turn to snort. They couldn't hear me say to myself, "For more reasons than one, I wish I were the Governor." And as a wistful afterthought, "I'm sure they sleep nights."

Babies and Midwives

[In 1934 the Dionne Quintuplets were born. The five identical sisters captured the world's attention, and continued to for many years, including that of the Thompson family.]

The difference between fame and comfortable obscurity may rest on so small a thing as presenting five brand new infants to ONE set of surprised parents, as opposed to five babies to FIVE sets of resigned parents. Jerry can apparently do no better than twins in spite of our Nancy's urging him on to Twin-triplets, as she calls them.

I am always astonished when I read about the alarming condition of the birth rate. It does so well by itself here, well enough to help adjust the balance in other less populous places and to keep us from getting away even for short vacations. Once in a long time, we snatch a day for ourselves between Mrs. B. and Mrs. S., just trusting to fate that Mrs. T. won't be early. But nearly always someone dies or has a bad heart attack or a baby, and we wish we hadn't gone. We leave with high hopes and keen anticipation and come home feeling that we have evaded our responsibilities.

The gradual change toward hospitalization has been a great boon to patient and doctor alike, but there are still many babies born at home for such reasons as:
    1. They think it is cheaper at home. But it isn't by the time they hire extra help and buy the necessary supplies.
    2. They are afraid of hospitals—Aunt Annie died in one.
    3. His mama and her mama had theirs at home.
    4. The babies might get mixed.

Early in his practice, when most of them arrived at home, Jerry had the assistance on many cases of a very capable colored midwife, Carrie. She used to say how sorry she felt for all doctors. "If I had to doctah as many wimin foh as many things as they does, I'd vomit when I looked at one of the creatures. The way them wimin folks follows them pore doctahs, you'd think they had sugah on they tails."

Jerry enjoyed Carrie. She managed her private affairs, as well as those of the small community where she lived. When her husband began to come home drunk and abusive, she waited until he was in a drunken stupor, then securely tied him up in a sheet and sat down to wait. When he awoke, more or less sober, she beat him up thoroughly, then loosed him from the sheet and served him a fine hot breakfast of all his favorite foods.

Once Carrie was the assistant when Mr. and Mrs. Joe New York were having a baby. He was called Joe New York because his name was unpronounceable, and because he was always comparing the mining settlement, where they were unfortunate enough to live, with New York City, where he spent a part of one day on his way from Hungary. Joe had obviously had too much to drink when Carrie arrived to take charge of the scene and heard him abusing his wife who was in labor. "Shet up you mouf, you," she ordered. The abusive language continued, the wife in tears. Carrie's wrath was beautiful to behold. "Put you foot where you mouf is at, you lazy good foh nothin'," she screamed, but instead Joe struck Mrs. Joe. Carrie rushed out into the kitchen and came back wielding a large bread knife, her eyes blazing. "NOW, will you get gone from heah?" Joe dashed out the door, Carrie at his heels. She continued to wave the knife as she chased him up over the hill to oblivion. The baby arrived without its papa. Joe sneaked in the back door after a twenty-four-hour absence, sober, chastened, and with a wary eye out for sturdy Carrie.

Busy evening office hours are very taxing for the Country Doctor after a long day, but they seem unavoidable. Many patients come in cars after Jerry is through work. There are always calls to make after office hours too.

I helped in the office one evening not long ago. I've forgotten all the patients except a three-month-old baby that had only gained a few ounces since birth. Its chest was hollow, its tummy very large. The skin was dry and the entire surface infected and sore. The mother was undernourished and listless. I asked her if she oiled the baby as routine care, and she looked surprised and answered in the negative. I gave her three sample bottles of baby oil and two tubes of cold cream, insisting that she begin regular care of the baby's skin as well as follow all the doctor's directions.

When the patients were all gone, Jerry asked me to go with him to make a call to see if I could keep him awake. The patient's baby was due and she was not feeling too well, so he wanted to check on her condition. They lived sixteen miles distant, so I asked if he thought there was any danger of its being necessary for him to stay. He thought not, so I went along, poorly clad for winter in a white silk dress, with no hat or gloves. While he was in the house, I sat in the car cutting an old coat of his into strips for a hooked rug background.

After quite a wait, he came out saying, "Sorry, but I'll have to go to the hospital at once, but I don't think I'll be very long." There was no opportunity for me to get home, so I went to the hospital and called some friends who picked me up and took me to their home. We sat waiting for Jerry until 2 A.M. then went to bed. Jerry came to break-fast and suggested that I go back in town to wait as he had ordered an X-ray, which would determine whether to put the patient at rest or operate. In either case, he could soon go home. This I was most anxious to do, not only because of my clothes, but because Nancy was in bed with swollen glands, and an insurance adjustor was due that morning.

The day was interminable. I knew that Aunt Lydia and Carrie, our older helper who had seen better times, would see that the house and Nancy were cared for. Carrie was super-efficient and quasi-melancholy. Every time I bought anything for the house or family, she would fold her arms, sigh deeply and say in a tone implying that she had just buried the last of her children, "I've wanted one of those all my life." I always felt guilty. I appreciated her efforts at economy but agreed with Nancy that when Carrie planned the meals, there was too much room left for water. I wanted to get home to see that they were not floating away! We left for home at 6 P.M. I had had no lunch as I did not wish to go out in such unsuitable clothing. Home has never looked more inviting. That evening he went out alone.

The same day that I read Karl Menninger in the February 1939 *Atlantic Monthly* and gathered the impression that all female ills could be solved by having babies and yet more babies, I accompanied Jerry out into the winter's worst blizzard. The snow was so heavy that he had to get out every few miles to assist the windshield wipers.

After about five miles on a main road, we turned off onto a dirt road and drove slowly until a crossroad loomed up, and in the snow, we could not see which fork to take. Jerry got out and shouted with volume that would have shamed Tarzan or the lady hog callers. Far off the right we heard a faint answer and saw the flicker of a lantern. The private lane was narrow and drifted, but we finally made it to the back door. The coal stove in the kitchen gave us a cheerful welcome.

The patient, who was having a baby, was in a downstairs room that contained two cribs beside her bed. I at first supposed that one was for the coming child, but a second glance showed that both were occupied. I judged that the babies were about two years and one. The mother looked to be seventeen and could not have been twenty, I am sure. Many of her teeth were missing. The two grandmothers were present, one had had sixteen grandchildren, and one twelve. I learned the details of all twenty-eight plus those of their immediate families. The one with twelve was the more talkative. One of her positive theories interested me, "You know what's wrong, these days? It's the auto. There is too many of them. It not only causes more pregnancies, but it is the cause of most of the trouble women has after they are pregnant. They go out jolting when they should be home working. I've had twelve. I never had no help. I washed, ironed, cooked, sewed, papered, scrubbed, whitewashed, milked eight cows, and did a thousand other things right up to when the babies come. And I never had no trouble. Women don't need hospitals. What they need is more work." Mussolini and Menninger would love her.

As the night wore on, both Jerry and I grew very tired. There was no place to rest. All the chairs had either holes in the seats or boards nailed across them. One chair and an old couch had such hilly springs that it was easier to stand. Our figures were too normal to adjust themselves. When I wasn't busy, I observed the works of art. On the mantel stood two plaster figures, one of Snow White and one of a Kewpie doll. A large framed picture of Shirley Temple beamed on the figures benevolently. Baby Stewart hung on the wall above a calendar.

I went out to the car to try to rest, but it was twenty degrees below zero, and the heater did not work, so I could not keep warm. When I returned to the scene of action, both children were awake studying proceedings until I persuaded a young sister-in-law to take them upstairs. She thought it would be too cold, but I wrapped one in a blanket and started so she followed suit.

About 2 A.M. someone suggested that there was coffee on the stove. Jerry and I nearly crashed the already decrepit furniture in our haste to reach the coffee. I found the largest cups in the kitchen and poured the black fluid from the old-fashioned coffee pot. With one sip, I gasped for air. It had boiled all day. Even in my condition, it was not to be endured and when it comes to coffee at 2 A.M., I'm no sissy. I carried the pot to the backyard and threw the contents as far as possible. I think they froze in mid-air. A search of the kitchen produced a familiar brand of coffee, so, with thanksgiving in my heart, I made a fresh pot of sixteen cups according to civilized standards. It revived both of us enough to see the night through with its arduous duties.

When all was over, we gathered up bags and wraps, and prepared to go. The lock on the car door was frozen. Matches did no good, so they carried hot water from the kitchen supply. When it was thawed out, the young father held the lantern and tried to direct our turning. The car skidded into a deep ditch. They lifted it out and we tried again. The windshield was solid ice under snow. Jerry got out an unnamed tool and scratched a small surface free. The other windows were completely covered. He had to get out repeatedly to scrape the window on the trip home. We were back at 5:30 A.M.

It was Nancy's birthday, so I got out the new doll clothes I had made and dressed the birthday doll as I warmed by the fire. I remember thinking that if I had just had that baby, I would then be resting. I laid the doll, Wendy Ann, on Nancy's pillow for her first surprise, then fell into bed.
Nancy had asked to be wakened at the exact minute she was eleven (1:30 A.M.), but at that hour we were ushering in another child to celebrate the same natal day.

That same evening Jerry was interrupted just as dinner was announced. He came back to the table and said, "I'll have to go. Do you want to go with me? Annie's in labor and you know she usually needs me quickly." I agreed to go and when Nancy asked me when we would be back, I said, "Soon, I hope, darling. Daddy's having a baby."

Aunt Lydia followed me out to the porch, gravely and hesitantly said, "I'm sure it is not wholesome for Nancy for you to be so frank." I was completely surprised.
"Why, Lydia, Nancy thinks no more of anyone having a baby than of a dental appointment. I wouldn't have her grow up with my youthful abnormal curiosity."
"Well, then, I must tell you what she told me the other day."—I expected the worst—She continued, "The other evening Nancy said, 'Aunt Lydia, if you ever start to grow a baby, don't think there is anything you can do about it. You'll just go ahead and have it when the time comes like any of the rest of us. I wonder how soon I'll have one?'"

I could see that Lydia was sincerely distressed, so promised to shush Nancy mildly for her benefit. It is really a problem. Howard and Nancy have our casual, normal viewpoint. Howard has greeted us when we came in late at night with the news that Mrs.——'s pains are five minutes apart, in much the same tone that he says, "I fixed the furnace and put Hitty to bed." And yet I heard Nancy say to a group of playmates, "My Daddy had a baby at the hospital last night." and soon they would have left her and be whispering behind a tree.

Life's experiment *The Birth of a Baby* interested me. Nancy came in after school and asked for *Life* as usual. I told her it was by her chair. She spent the usual time looking and reading, then laid it down and said to me, "Well, I guess I'll go and play with my dolls. Don't miss *Life* this week. It has some awful interesting pictures about a baby getting born." So maybe I am right. At least Nancy will never help to organize a club called F.O.A.B.—Find Out About Babies—as I once did. Even at a tender age, I didn't believe the brothers who told me that the mother opened up like the Red Sea, and just as miraculously closed again.

After reassuring Lydia, we hurried to Annie. I had helped with several of her babies. They are a special colored family (so many are!). The husband brings us a dressed hog in the winter and plows our garden in the Spring. To reciprocate, we help with that year's baby. Nancy sorts out enough playthings to furnish the family with a complete Christmas every year, and since there are eight children, this means real generosity on her part as she inherits the cursed trait of wanting to treasure everything. You should see our attic. It would explain ancestor worship. Once in a while I find a timid little moth and wonder what generation it is.

As we approached the weather-beaten shack, it looked like a beehive with children of all ages buzzing about. We arrived just in time to welcome Annie's sweet new baby, and before we left, we heard her proclaimed Lelia Cornelia Mardoree Spurlock.

As we drew up in front of the hospital one evening, Jerry asked me to call on Mrs. R. Going up the steps he said, "For heaven's sake don't wear that mangey fur coat while you are in here. I can't stand it." "But darling," I protested, "the lapels look lovely and I have learned to face the public as I gracefully back out of any situation, and to carry my elbows pointed in. It hasn't been easy to acquire." However,

I saw that he was suffering, so removed the coat, and chilled as I went into the air-conditioned elevator, carrying best pelts forward. I gave my old brown velvet dress an extra hitch, (it acted better the first time it was made over) and went to call on his patient.

Jerry nearly had apoplexy when the patient said to a caller, "Well, he certainly does dress her well." And my mood matched his when the patient said, "Doctor, I think you'd better sign me out a day or two early. My husband is helping the hired girl with the dishes. That isn't like him."

Among other minor lessons I have learned as the wife of the country doctor, is not to accompany him a la nightgown. One summer night I pulled a top coat over my nightie and went along for the ride. At 7 A.M. I sat rigidly on the front seat and tried not to acknowledge to myself the tantalizing odors of bacon and coffee which came from the open window. When I was cordially invited in, I smiled as warmly as I could and said, "Thank you so much, but I never eat breakfast." I have never thought a doctor's wife would be held accountable for untruths, the bookkeeping would be too complicated.

On another night a former college friend of mine was visiting us and we were ready for bed when Jerry was called out. He dared us to go along, so we added rather frothy negligees and mules and went. Someplace in No Man's Land, the car stalled in the mud. I offer, as a novel experience, trying to help get a car out of heavy mud, shod in mule. The word in singular form is indicated.

My mental library has a shelf stacked with interesting cases. Once I helped Jerry on a lengthy case many miles off the beaten track. I entertained a spoiled child, rode horseback to a neighbor's, cleaned two chickens for the family larder, prepared a meal, helped the doctor, oiled the new baby, and was rewarded by a namesake. The mother thought my name sounded like a movie show.

One of the novel cases was a woman in labor who drank a quart of straight whiskey (she was fairly well conditioned for it) before she called Jerry. She had three pairs of shoes under the bed and every time her anxious spouse would climb the stairs to offer assistance, she would reach for a shoe and hurl it at him with unpleasant accusations. I remembered a midwife's admonition that a hatchet under the bed would cut the pains, and thought it was well that the patient confined her weapons to shoes.

The details of one Sunday are graven on my memory. From 4 P.M. to 4 A.M. we had four guests to tea, made five calls, went to the hospital where Jerry saw several patients, stopped at the home of a friend to call. The phone rang, calling Jerry home. We averaged fifty-five miles an hour. Grabbed our bags at the office and dashed to a nearby town.

The nurse on the job was an elderly lady who had never seen a birth. In spite of a raging headache, I helped all I could. When I opened the box of supplies, I discovered no silver nitrate for the baby's eyes. It necessitated a six-mile dash to rouse the druggist from sleep. Back and I discovered that the nurse could not care for the new baby, so I began to oil it very sketchily, using the kitchen table for support. My head was bursting, and I was sick with nausea. Jerry came and completed the task which he thought I was doing too slowly. I dragged myself outside to relieve my sick stomach.

At 3:45 A.M. en route home, both dead tired, Jerry said, "You know, my love, I believe you are too fastidious for this game." I had no stiletto, so lowered the window for more air! No, Jerry's never had quintuplets, but among other multiples have been: Mixed Twins, Flossie and Fleesie, Unmixed Twins, Virgin and Mary, and the Gold Dust Runners-up, whose care he relished, Damon Paul and Pythias Saul.

The Counry Doctor's Wife Entertains

Even the thought of entertaining gives me a slight chill of apprehension but nevertheless, we love company and try it often. The
strenuous years have made shabby spots in the house in spite of mild
efforts at rehabilitation and some of the rugs are down to the tread,
but I dim the lights, ask more people to come and rugs don't show.

I can remember no occasion when Jerry was not interrupted at
least once. There have been times without number when he has not
appeared on the horizon at all, but more often he is in the throes of
dressing when guests arrive and manages to have a few minutes as
host before being called away. Fortunately, his personality is vibrant
enough to cast an aura which envelops us during his absence.

If dinner is announced before he leaves, his few minutes are frequently spent entertaining guests by whetting the carving knife with great
vim and vigor. The task amounts to a greater passion with him. It is
never done previous to the arrival of the guests but always after dinner is announced. He gets a gleam in his eye and rushes at the carving
set. He asks for the steel, begins a rhythmic motion, and I imagine I
see his lips counting. He prides himself on the rhythm—just a carving
knife jitter bug at heart! The act should, by all means, be accompanied
by stirring music, preferably Wagner. The roast, or what have you, is
gradually cooling. He tries the knife, it does not cut him, so he rises
from the table, even if we have white-coated the pseudo-gardener for
a little local color, and repairs to the kitchen where he hopes to find
an emery stone.

Conversation is somewhat stilted during his kitchen sojourn. My
saliva begins to dry up, my thoughts to flow more rapidly. This is

one endurance test not foreseen in marriage vows. He returns with a smile of satisfaction on his face and takes up the fork to begin carving. It is here that the door or telephone bell usually rings and he excuses himself.

We do not carry guest liability, so I try to carry on, feeling it is too much to ask a guest to take charge of the dangerous weapon. It would split a hair before he begins the sharpening act.

Gentle reader, if you have a husband who does not sharpen the knife after you are assembled at the table, hang on to him like grim death, he is the only one extant. During each event, I resolve thereafter to have friends to tea or to prepare canned salmon in gala dress, but I am a good wife and I want him to be happy, so on he whets, and on we go with serving rolled roasts, thick steaks, or a crown roast of lamb.

There are two sides to all these major issues. I recently heard him tell a bridegroom when admiring a Sterling carving set, that it only required about ten years to get a carving knife on the table that would cut. As I eavesdropped, I was reminded of the friend who said to me, "But they require managing, my dear. I've used a teaspoonful of tact here and a teaspoon there, and in seven years, I have a new house."

When the inevitable call comes by telephone, sometimes I answer and if my reliable intuition senses it is not urgent, I lie with a clear conscience, but when the call is at the front door, they see him basking in the candlelight. The house was not designed for subterfuge. The car is never put in the garage, so it flaunts itself like the President's flag when the Doctor is in residence. Fortunately, our friends understand and are entertained by the hectic condition of our household.

Last summer I planned a super picnic. Susie and I spent hours making sandwiches and salad. It all began propitiously. Jerry came promptly and we had no patients waiting. This presaged ill. We packed up the supper and left quickly before a call might interfere.

When we arrived at the beautiful woods, we parked the car near
the highway, wandered down among the trees, and built a huge fire.
When we left home, we had not given a forwarding address but
somehow, someway, we were tracked down. A man called Jerry outside the charmed circle. He was evidently persuasive, as Jerry excused
himself to be gone 'Just a few minutes—long enough to give the fire
a burning start.' We relaxed and enjoyed the soft shadows and the
designs made by the showers of sparks. For a time the stories and
strange harmonies were great fun, but when I suddenly woke to the
realization that all the food was in the car with Public Enemy No. 1,
things began to sound a trifle forced.

Time wore on, the fire passed to ashes, there was no sound of a
leaping motor car. At long last, we left the dying embers to a hoot-
ing owl--embers that exuded no tantalizing odor of sizzled steaks.
Homeward wended, we our weary ways with our tails between our
legs and our tongues hanging out. I slept fitfully and dreamed that I
was starving in the midst of plenty.
Bright and early the next morning, Jerry dragged himself into the
house carrying baskets and packages. For the first time, it dawned on
me that his naturally rugged and cheerful features could relax into an
expression of futility. Waffles and sausage restored him. We ate steak
for a week. But I can't complain too much. Once we actually had a
party without a single interruption for several days.

The roads in those days were not cleared of snow until nature took a
hand. Now alas, they are kept open, thanks to hot-mix or cold-poli-
tics. Our house party of eight guests arrived in a blinding snowstorm
and were the last persons to enter town for five days. With helpers,
Jerry shoveled them in from this end while they worked from the
other. We had expected them to stay from Friday to Monday and
had laid in a large supply of food accordingly. We were completely
snowed in, telephone wires down, drifts eight feet high. No bread
or mail entered the village. When Monday came, the roads were still
blocked. It was wonderful. Jerry had never spent so much time at
home since we were married. He was the superb host with leisure
to employ his talents. We had one grand session after another, great

talks by the fire, (Isn't it amazing how few are the people to whom conversation is an art)? And even a little theater with original offerings and doubtful talent. We slept and ate when we felt like it.

Late Monday evening our bridge game was interrupted by a great tramping out front. At the curb stood two bedraggled nags, doing their best to stand up under the weight of their saddles. One sagged appreciably when he sighted Jerry! The man on the porch had come to ask Jerry to make a trip about seven miles out in the country over a road barely passable in summer. His wife was having a baby and he had been so long en route to our house that he felt desperate. When questioned about the condition of the road, he said, "Oh, you can't get through the road before Spring. I came out fence rows and through the fields."

We helped Jerry get ready and saw them off. The next morning we were all up street on a sort of treasure hunt trying to assemble food, canned or otherwise, when we saw a caravan approaching. I shall not soon forget the sight. The Country Doctor, all 225 pounds of him, covered with snow and muffled to the ears, (the patient's family had pulled a long woolen stocking over his head) sat astride a dingy white horse so fat and with such middle-aged spread that the Doctor's tired legs stuck out at right angles. I was afraid to inquire about the previous two horses. Near each leg dangled a Boston bag, slightly the worse for wear. (I never see a Boston bag [two-handled bag for carrying books, etc.] that I don't remember that Nancy chose to carry dancing slippers in a paper sack saying, "I don't like to carry that black bag, I'm no obstetric.").
In hilarious mood, nine of us formed a court of honor to see the caravan home. Two generous guests offered shoulder supports for the right-angled limbs but were refused in language unbecoming in a host. For a week afterward, Jerry would wake from a nightmare in which he thought he was still astride that broad-beamed mare.

A New Year's party stands out vividly in our memories. When Jerry was dressing, he said, "It is never safe to put on these glad rags—something is sure to happen."

The first call came about a half-hour after our friends had assembled. I took his hand at bridge and the room was fairly quiet when the front door burst open and a wild-eyed man rushed in. With loud voice, he shouted, "I'm dying! Help me! I haven't breathed for ten minutes." The party as one man was stricken dumb and sat paralyzed. I took his arm and persuaded him to lie down on the davenport, pulling one of the pillows out so his head would be lowered. I could observe that he was breathing but sent one of the boys after Jerry, bathed the face and hands of the patient with cold water, and kept him quiet until Jerry came and took him home. While they were gone, the phone rang.

I answered and heard an excited youthful voice, "Tell the Doctor to come over to our place right away. We live three miles beyond Shady Hill school. I've just shot my Dad. And ask Doc to call the sheriff before he comes. I'll be waitin' on the road."

I called the sheriff, and Jerry left as soon as he returned from seeing 'Nellie' home. He was gone for a long time and had a weird experience to report when he returned. He was driving down a lonesome single-track road, almost impassable because of rocky ledges, when suddenly a figure stepped out of the shadow flashing a strong light. He carried a large automatic gun, and Jerry was, of course, not armed so he slowed down, stiff with fright. It proved to be the boy who had called. "For God's sake, Doc, put out those lights. I took a crack at my old man, but if he is still alive, he'll kill us sure."

Jerry turned out his lights with alacrity and tried backing his car in the dark, having lost any desire to drive farther. In a short time, the officers arrived, and the boy volunteered to show them how to approach the house so his father couldn't see them. They surrounded the house cautiously and from a point on a higher level threw a strong searchlight on the little shack. The light silhouetted a figure slumped in a chair with head fallen forward on a table. The 15-year-old sighed with relief, "Thank God, I got him. Now I'm ready to go with you, Sheriff, if you will let me tell my mother."

They all went down to the house. The man still clutched a gun in his inert hand. He was unshaven and slovenly in dress and had a sinister expression on his face. In the center of his forehead was a blood-clotted hole. The boy had shot first when he saw his father's threatening gesture. The man had abused his family for years. All of them had left home except the mother, a young baby, and this lad who was afraid to leave her to the mercies of his father.

That evening she, with her baby, had fled in terror to a neighbor's house, and the son decided to take things in his own hands. He entered the house to try to persuade his father to leave home but carried his gun because he knew his father was armed.

After the post mortem, Jerry came in just as Aurora ushered in the light of a new year. The white bosom of his dress shirt was blood-stained, and his collar was missing. When he had relaxed for a few minutes, I volunteered the information that Rosie, our kitchen in-cumbent of the moment was not yet in.

Now Rosie was a joy. She could cook and she loved it. She was clean and happy. She loved us all, but she loved dance marathons more. She had been coming in at daylight. The neighbors were worrying about her morals. I had remonstrated gently, and she had promised to do better as she really wanted to stay. Jerry looked out and saw the car down the street several doors. He became volubly impatient. He donned his best overcoat and his stiff hat and stalked out with great dignity, dress clothes and all. I did not ask his intentions, feeling sure they were honorable, but kept watch from a dim recess on the porch.

He approached the car. It was standing at the foot of a slope. He called—no answer—and started down to the car. A loud crash ac-companied by vigorous words followed. He had slipped on the ice and his hat careened into the street. The crash awoke the occupants. It had not improved Jerry's disposition, but, hatless he mustered what aplomb he could and invited her in for her things. I never have a camera at the right moments.

She left in the dawn of the new year, but she liked us so much that she called Jerry when she had her first baby. As we wearily climbed the stairs that January first, Jerry smiled a bit crookedly and said, "Nice New Year's party."

A recent dinner party sounds too fantastic to have happened. We had four guests and dinner had begun without accident or incident. The carving knife was sharpened. My hopeful wish that the peaceful beginning might continue was interrupted by the telephone Jerry answered and promised to go at once. He hung up the receiver and said that someone had beaten up his wife and fractured her arm.

It was in a small town only a few miles away, so we [she and their dinner guests] decided to go with him. We had a mad ride up and down a succession of hills. After he had been in the house for a few minutes, he called me. Six wild-eyed children were ranged along the wall of the room where their mother lay on the bed. Jerry asked me to take the small baby from the bed and entertain all the children in the other room. (Someday a nightclub or two is going to waken to my possibilities. I can entertain anything from a sick dog to a man with D.T's and both seem to frequent such places. My shoulders aren't so bad either.)

It was difficult not to overhear the conversation in the next room since the patient was excited and in pain. One of the boys added an illuminating detail, "Mom came home and found Pop in bed with Angela. Mom didn't seem to like it and when she said sompin', Pop slugged her." Pop was somewhat chastened by the time of our arrival and Angela was not among those present. Pop offered us all kinds of bottled beverages. He was generous and expansive telling Annie, "I'll get you that new dress tomorrow—maybe, yes? Annie?"

Jerry set the broken arm and the newly devoted husband agreed to take her for an X-ray the following morning. When she was quiet and comfortable, we returned to our salads.
We had been seated all of five minutes when there were hurried steps on the porch. An excited father begged Jerry to come at once as his baby had a fever of 105 degrees and they thought it was dying. Jerry said, "Come on," so out we, and our guests, dashed again. The baby was ill of pneumonia. The room temperature was 94 degrees, and the mother was exhausted from day and night care of the sick baby for five days. She feared fresh air or a bath for the baby.

Jerry told them he would ask the druggist to send over some medicine. The father replied, "I have a little money, Doc, but if you're going to send the druggist, I'd better save the money for him. And say Doc, could you bring over a bottle of consecrated cod liver oil tomorry when you come?" It would not take an Edgar Hoover to wonder why he didn't want the druggist to bring it.

Back home for dessert. Halfway through the ice cream, someone pounded vigorously on the front door, and we hear an excited voice, "Come quick, Doctor. My sister has tried to commit suicide."

He asked us if we wanted to go this time and we agreed to see it through. It was a faster trip than the others. (A dealer in automobiles, or a manufacturer whose car will stand up to Jerry's driving, should be happy to furnish us cars free, for the advertising. Any car that can stand up to that pressure has something). As we drew near the house, we could sense the excitement. Instead of stopping in front of the house, Jerry drove in the driveway and around to the back of the house. The lights of the car showed an old barn with a door slightly ajar and a rope was dangling from a hidden timber. But the thing that sent shivers down our spines was the printing in large red letters on the face of the old barn,

> HE WHO ENTERS
> HERE LEAVES
> HOPE BEHIND

Jerry was gone for a long time and we had little desire for conversation in the car. I thought and hoped that the delay indicated a favorable prognosis. It did. We came home seeking lots of black coffee and long intervals of heavenly silence.

At Susie's urgent invitation, we took some friends to the colored camp meeting which is the highlight of the year socially and emotionally for the colored community. She wanted us to go that particular Sunday after the Big Storm for they would all be out professing a change of heart so another storm wouldn't get them. "But I can't blame them. I was so scared that I tasted it on my tongue and I saw trees blown down in the cemetery when so many of them there needs shade."

The meeting was held outdoors in a grove of trees. Hundreds of people attended. There was preaching all day, and the audience came and went at will. I leaned against a wagon wheel to hear an afternoon sermon. The text was announced in sonorous tones, "The wedges of sin is death. There is all kinds of sinners, my brethren and sisters. I've been hearing lots of mutterings about who is going to preach at camp meetin' tonight. Well, I'll tell you who's goin' to preach—I'm goin' to preach, and stop chewin your teeth and sayin' to yourself 'I can hear him any time, too much'. Unruffle your feathers, you complainin' sinners, I can see you all any time, too, too much. Tonight I'm goin' to preach about what sisters has enough religion to have control of their children, judgin' by how many of their children stays to church, and how many insults the Lord by chewin' gum."

He continued, "How many of you is backslid? You are convert-ed —you sin again. You try to get back. It's never the same. It's like when you have a daughter who marries, disagrees with her husband, and comes home to live. It's never the same. The wedges of sin is death—they has got her. You can't tell her what to do anymore. She knows as much as you do." We stayed until the last wedge.

Most of the audience looked pretty subdued until the singing of spirituals began. Then they all woke up and thoroughly forgot the threats hanging over their heads. After the song, Sister Josie was asked to close the session with prayer. Susie says that Sister would flip her tail up over her back if she had a tail. She arose from her hard bench and flipped up to the front, rolled her eyes solemnly, and then knelt to pray. She began, "Oh, Good Lord Jesus" and raised her head slightly to study the effect of her beginning. A wasp, which had been attending service more through curiosity than a desire to worship, entered the neck of her black silk blouse. She arose like Ferdinand—without flipping—and the meeting adjourned sans benediction. As we walked to our car, Jerry was stopped many times

Cornelia Cattell Thompson

to answer questions or to admire offspring, frequently namesakes. One man called him aside, "Doctor, could you please give me a few big words. I have to take charge of experience meetin' tonight and I wants to show a little learnin'." I heard Jerry suggest **idiosyncrasy, hyperbole, procrastination.**

Later, when the minister came to speak to us, we spoke of our pleasure in the meeting. Susie interrupted, "It was all right, Reverend, but you preached too long. I've got spiritual indigestion."
A rain which had been brewing, burst on us and Susie's indigestion. We and our guests hurried to our car. There was no shelter for most of the zealots. They stood huddled in groups like chickens in the rain, not ducks which proverbially shed water. None departed. Camp meeting day is not one to be dismissed lightly because of rain. I knew their feathers would soon fluff up when the sun came out.

Our guests agreed with us that we were all decidedly refreshed. Jerry and I resolved to do more of our entertaining away from home. It offers unusual diversion and less interruption.

I Wouldn't Change It If I Could

A favorite professor of mine was a learned woman under whom I imbibed not only French Literature of the seventeenth century but many of her livable philosophical observations as well. In rapid French, not always understood by the majority of her pupils, she would talk off her exasperation with the indifference of her students—a fitting subject—as she fixed her gaze at some distant point on the campus.

"They say that youth is the time of joy. It is not so. The joys and sorrows of youth are of too great intensity." And then reluctantly dragging back her attention to the inattentive class before her, she would break into emphatic English. "Youth is shallow, it is vain, it is selfish and not tempered with the wisdom of experience. I would not be young again."

I wonder if she feels the same today. After her retirement, her small savings were dissipated during bank and real estate failures, and her living standards were of necessity greatly curtailed. I was for a time able to sell enough silhouettes which she imported from Germany, to pay some of her necessary expenses, but not enough to be of permanent benefit.

Her words have recurred to me times without number when I have experienced an appreciation of some event or conversation not possible in my adolescent years. When Nancy asked me, "Don't you wish you could grow down to a little girl again?" I assured her that I like being grown up, at least enough to be her mother. I doubt too if when very young I could appreciate so keenly Nancy's names for two of Hitty's puppies, Grapes and Wrath.

There is so much I would remember, every type of experience from the little boy who wanted to give all the pennies in his bank to Jerry in return for the new baby and only sister just presented to a large family of boys, to the smell of burning flesh when an elderly lady, who had fallen into an open fire, held up burned arms from which the flesh hung in scorched ribbons exposing the bones and begged to be allowed to die.

If it were all tragic, it could not be endured, but there is constant change from tragedy to light comedy. One minute, it is a little baby with Down Syndrome, and the next, the patient will be an elderly man who has walked out to the office to see if Jerry will find someone to sit up with him that night, as he thinks he is developing "walking typhoid fever"—he wants to walk all the time.

The parents of the former youth are exhausted from financial and emotional worry, and perhaps Jerry will be the fifth or sixth M.D. consulted as desperate hope urges them on from one doctor to another. It is difficult to tell them that the facial characteristics and listless expression indicate mental deficiency, but a conscientious doctor, in this case at least, believes quick truth is the greatest kindness.

The latter case is easier to handle and less wearing on the emotions. What the village lacks in Empire State Buildings and Arnold Arboretums, it makes up for in character types. The walking typhoid fever prospect is the ineptly verbose type. He pushes aside the straggling remnants of a drooping mustache and wheedles Jerry, "Doc, kin you give me an autopsy of my symptoms for about two bits? I think I've been ridin' too much in my son's new Ford cafeteria and I ain' t feelin' myself." But the few minutes of social intercourse and flattering attention send him on his way recovered from one imaginary ailment and ready with a new day to scout for another.

Another emotion was called into play the day I answered the doorbell and found myself face to face with a man covered with smallpox sores. I urged him to go home quickly and promised to send the doctor. Never have I scrubbed so long or so viciously. Jerry was not here to consult, so the doorbell, the door frame, the entire front porch became for a time my mortal enemy and were attacked with a procession of laundry soap, ammonia, kerosene, scouring powder, carbolic acid, and Lysol. I acted on Solomon's principle that if a little will do good, more will do better. He adds salt and turpentine to an old wives mixture of red pepper and gasoline to treat almost anything. If I had known then, about the gasoline and red pepper, I'd probably have been siphoning a patient's car. The patient's face is still pock-marked. Due to kind Fate or much scrubbing, ours are not.

One particularly dark night I was trying to read in the car which was quite a distance from the house where Jerry was calling. An elderly lady came out to the car. "Won't you come into the warm kitchen with me? I think the doctor will be here a good while because Sam's baby's having convulsions."
I thanked her and went in. I helped with the dishes while we discussed things of common interest: dishwashing, housekeeping, cooking, with an exchange of favorite recipes, sick children, gardening. She had no teeth, her hair was a dull iron-gray, thin and straggly, her figure drooped in strategic places, her hands were worn and red, but she was so clean, so cheerfully philosophical, and had such natural kindliness that I remember the evening and the conversation in detail.
She said, "Some women fuss and pretend they don't like to keep house and cook and have babies, but, you know, I don't believe them? There's something in us women that makes us happy inside when we keep busy at everyday things, and the inside matters more than the outside. I believe the reason I worry more about my grandchildren when they are sick than I did about my own, is because I was too busy then to stop for a good worry." I asked about the size of her family. "I have fourteen, and the last one came six months after my husband died with pneumonia." I found a suitable reply difficult, but she sighed and continued, "At first, I thought I couldn' t live without John but—it's been a good life. It wasn' t so hard after I made up my mind to just do it."

If I were the motto-type, I'd hang that in the kitchen.

Numerous conversations and happenings brighten most days.
Occasionally the humor is not appreciated to the fullest until viewed
in retrospect. In the days when gasoline stations were not so plentiful, and when the level of the gasoline in the tank plus the degree of
the slope determined whether the hill was negotiable, we started up
a winding two mile hill on a dark rainy night.

The motor sputtered, the car stopped. Jerry managed one of his
miraculous turns and we tried going up backward. This often solved
the difficulty but not on this rainy night. He got out and made some
cursory examinations and reported, "Out of gas." I did not wish
to sit in the car at 1 A.M. on a lonesome road while he walked back
to the nearest small town so I offered my services to a very tired
Country Doctor. We found two fat medical magazines in the car,
and these opened, served as combination hat and umbrella.

After splashing along for about a mile, we roused the occupants of
a small shack which boasted one unlighted gasoline pump in front.
An elderly man in trousers and nightshirt found an old pail which
he filled with gasoline. Jerry tied a newspaper over the top, thanked,
and paid the man, who waved us off, "Sorry folks, I ain't got a car to
take you back. Jest keep the bucket."

Back we trudged, Jerry, carrying a splashing pail with one hand and
steadying the Journal of The American Medical Association on his
head with the other. Their ultimate destination is not usually so util-
itarian. I held a journal of some other brand with one hand and my
nose with the other, for the fumes from Jerry's burden were mingled
with those left when a skunk had preceded us. When we reached the
car, I held the otoscope, in lieu of a flashlight, while he poured gasoline through an improvised paper funnel, then with an airy gesture
tossed the bucket over the hill.

Dripping and shivering we piled into the car. He turned the key and
stepped on the starter. Nothing happened. Again. Nothing. With
a sigh that shook the car, he got out for further investigation. He
pointed to a stream of liquid, unlike rain. He had forgotten to close

the petcock on the carburetor. Bolstered with good intuition, I can anticipate and forestall many catastrophes, but petcocks, whatever they are, are out of my line, and in a class with plumbing. The gas ran merrily down the hill and so did we, with a change of adverbs and the addition of expletives, but not before a devilish search in brambles for an old bucket, search personally conducted by me. Jerry says he's allergic!

Tired from being out most of that night, Jerry was called from break-fast, the one calling saying excitedly, "Someone shot." He finished his coffee and dashed out. At lunch, he told us that a little girl had been playing with other children under a grape arbor. A neighbor sat near cleaning his gun and talking with her father. Suddenly a shot rang out and the little girl fell. In a few minutes she was dead, the neighbor deeply remorseful. (How many times have I heard Father say, "It's the unloaded gun that does the damage?") I went to sympathize with the grieving mother. She thanked me and said, "Yes, isn't it dreadful, but we have to give her up so I tell Jim, let's get it over with as soon as possible. He didn't mean to do it but if he had been uptown loafing with the men like he should have been, this wouldn't have happened."

Sometimes amusing incidents are purely personal and have nothing to do with our dear public, which has such an insidious way of entering all phases of our experiences. There was the time when, after months of illness, I had been brought home from the hospital in a cast. It had seemed to be the last resort in efforts to treat a bad back. Weeks of lying with table boards in the bed had not relieved the condition. And do let me add, it is the perfect way to reduce. Just have a good heavy cast installed in summer, and you will melt away with no volition of your own. And if you have modernistic aspirations, the bi-valved cast, after its immediate purpose is fulfilled, might make an unusual stan-dard for a birdbath in the garden.

The turn of our stairway is short and I am long. Just then I could not bend, and since it seemed unfitting to upend me like a mummy, I was deposited on a hospital bed downstairs. The entire household, barring the invalid, bustled around to prepare for the coming of my brother and his family from Boston. We were well supplied with help.

One who had previously lived with us returned to act as a sympathetic and competent nurse. In the kitchen, we had Edna, who was sent from the city by a fond auntie. She was to be a rare find, the southern mammy type. We never saw her smile. She dyed the gravy with vegetable coloring. She couldn't read, and on this busy day, she decorated two rolls of canned dog food with parsley and placed them before a surprised family for lunch. I had ordered canned fish. When I remonstrated, she said it smelled better than salmon or tuna. There was no answer to that.

She talked aloud to herself all that day as she worked and seemed to be having queer hallucinations. She tied a fresh apron around her expansive middle and answered the door with the query, "Has you-all got a caird to leave foh the doctah?" This left the unsuspecting patient at a complete loss for words as leaving cairds just isn't done in these here parts.

It was a definite drawback to discover also that she was insane. As soon as we could arrange it, we dropped her off in her city, ostensibly for a short vacation. I knew perfectly well that she had all her worldly possessions with her, and that she had no intention of returning to this countryside where she privately referred to the natives as Cann-I-belles. And she knew too, that I had no intention of having her return. Our beautifully polite conversation at parting was classic. She gave me her address in case I needed her before the vacation ended. She hoped I would not overdo it.

Every square inch of the house was thoroughly combed and massaged and made to look its best. They arrived at the specified time, chatted a few minutes and all sat down in the living room. Howard and young Dickie were tussling, cub fashion, on the davenport. About one minute later there was a loud crash. Fifteen square feet of the ceiling fell on all the guests, leaving me who was carefully insulated against shock, untouched. There were no serious casualties but many scratches and bruises. It was a dusty greeting worthy of Mack Sennett [father of American slapstick comedy].

Jerry asked me to make a call with him one beautiful Spring morning. There was the first special green in the fields; small streams had taken on fresh life. I stopped to gather white wood violets. We drove slowly to enjoy it. On a narrow country road, a speeding car pushed us over on loose stone and our car, having too little momentum for once in its life, lost its balance and turned completely over. We sat stunned for several seconds, then awkwardly crawled out through the window, Jerry's cigarette still intact. We laughed when we discovered no broken bones and that both doors would open.

The course of destiny of finances both individual and national during the past decade makes one stop to ponder what course to pursue. I recall a memorable object lesson. One night Jerry was called about 1:30 A.M. to see a sick baby some distance from here. He tried to make some inquiries about the case, but all he could learn was that the baby was very sick. They said they had no doctor.

I went along to save him time as I knew the location of the house. We found two generations of a family pacing the floor with great anxiety. A very new baby lay twitching with convulsions. The mother was still in bed and trying to make the tiny child comfortable. They explained to Jerry that because of dissatisfaction they had paid and dismissed the doctor who had been in charge of the case.
After examination and observation, Jerry told them he thought the baby was dying from a cerebral hemorrhage. An experienced practical nurse later called him aside and said in a scared whisper, "I've seen a lot of these cases, Doctor, but I never before saw a Doctor get up and use his knees on the woman's abdomen to add pressure when the baby was slow coming."

Downstairs the garrulous and grief-stricken grandfather kept moaning, "I'm a self-made man. I have saved and scrimped all my life so I would have money and time for leisure when I was old. I've worked so hard I'm a broken old man. My five children are all grown and don't need me. All I want is to enjoy life with my grandchild. What good is my money when my only grandchild is dying?" We watched with him while his hope died.

Jerry made a call at an abandoned-looking farmhouse one evening at dusk. We had trouble getting in the muddy lane, which was not kept in repair because the farm tenants had no car. An elderly man and a wisp of a wife lived alone. She came out to talk to me. "It surely is nice to see someone to talk to," she said. "It gets pretty lonesome, just Frank and me and now he's sick, I have to do all the outside work too." She was carrying a quart bottle of milk and when I inquired about it, her reply sobered me. "I take this every morning and night to a neighbor up the road about a mile and I get eight cents for it. I hate to leave, but I guess I'd better excuse myself and run along so I'll get back to Frank before dark. He gets lonesome."

The doorbell rang one evening recently and a colored patient of long-standing asked Jerry if he could come over to the office. His heart sank, for he anticipated another baby, with others in the family not yet paid for. He went over. The wife sat in the reception room. She smiled and asked, "How much money do we owe you, Doc?" Jerry looked up the balance and gave it to them casually and without hope. They further astonished him. "How much will you take to settle the whole bill?" Jerry gasped and made a substantial reduction of the total amount with a mental reservation that he hadn't expected five dollars. The woman replied, "That's fair enough," and unrolled enough bills to pay in full. She had hit the numbers after playing a dream number. My Quaker childhood training would have called that tainted money, but Jerry's was fortunately different.

Occasionally we run across inescapable evidences of unscrupulous M.D.'s —shades of the proverbial brotherhood ethics. (I'll be black-mailed 'for admitting such heresy.) I watched Jerry with ill-concealed venom tear in two a check from a fellow doctor who appreciated so much the patient recently sent to him that he feels he must show some concrete evidence of same! He returned the torn pieces. I have never understood professional ethics in the practice of medicine and how it got that way. I suppose it is unreasonable of me to wonder why Jerry, who sees a patient several times and makes a correct diagnosis, receives six dollars on the books, and the surgeon receives one hundred and fifty in cash. It has puzzled countless others, so I'll not worry about it. But I'm not permitted to think this, least of all to express it. I merely whisper.

From my layman's viewpoint, a worse scoundrel than the aforementioned fee splitter is the doctor who would hold out false hope. One night I saw a desolate home, bare of even the crudest essentials. A tired mother held an imbecile child of about five years. She had given all her strength and spent every cent she could accumulate with doctors who held out hope of a cure. Jerry told her to face the truth that nothing could be done for her child but told her how to contact the county health authorities who would take her and her baby for further investigation. He then urged the mother to go at once for treatment of a face cancer. She was worn to the point of exhaustion.
"But Doctor, we have nothing left. We have spent over $4,000, all our life savings, on our baby and even sold our furniture and farm animals. I can't even pay you."

We drove the twelve miles home very quietly. On nights like that, it is hard to sleep. The most difficult phase of our work is to see so much real need, for medical services and for physical needs, and yet be unable to alleviate the condition due to limited income.

Shortly after I had been released from my cast—I was sleeping in it like an oyster on the half shell—I had an interesting caller. An elderly patient asked if she could come in and wait for the doctor as she was in great pain. Of course, I urged her to stay and I have never been sorry. I have many a quiet chuckle over that visit. The first amusing conversation occurred after the young practical nurse had answered the doorbell and had been unsuccessful in dismissing two inebriated patients at the door. With difficulty I managed, by leaning on a cane and holding on to various pieces of furniture, to make it to the door.

My personality got through. Soon they shuffled off the porch. When I turned back, my caller asked cheerfully, "Do you think you will ever walk right again?"

"Why, yes, I am hoping to, and the doctors tell me I will."

"Well, don't let them kid you. I know the signs and you won't ever walk right again."

The conversation went merrily on in this vein, mostly one-sided and in question form. I added enough sparks to keep it from dying out. "Do you think Parson's house burned down all by itself?" (Pregnant pause) "Doesn't that sound pretty funny to you?" (P.P.) She required no answers.

"Do you think Mrs. James poisoned herself?" (PP) How'd she get it? (Longer P.P.) And finally, she leaned forward and half-whispered, "Are you ever jealous?"

"No, I don't believe so. At least I try not to be."

"I'm not either. I always say there's plenty more I could get."

I studied her more closely. She was sans teeth and nearly sans hair. Her features jutted. I saw no evidence of pain or beauty. As she chattered, her pointed chin working up and down like a marionette's, I mused that after all, Beauty must not be skin deep but a figment of a rosy-tinted imagination.

She continued, "You say you don't wonder what he's doing when he's away?"

"Well, no, I don't. I know he is usually pretty busy. But would you advise me to?"

A tone of dark suspicion crept in, "Well, I'm not so sure. None of them can be trusted. You say he's been out since supper?"

"But his car is new and he must drive slowly."

"Four hours? Seven miles? (P. P.) Figure it for yourself."

I did. It didn't make sense!

I am not one of the ten best-dressed women, but I know a church sister who refused the bread of communion because she was on a diet. I know an old man who attributes his longevity to his strength of character in resisting onions and tobacco, alcohol not mentioned. He is saturated with both. I know an elderly spinster who was too nice to be catheterized, but after two days, had a change of heart to save her bladder.

I know one who cheerfully accepts financial straits by pear boiling side meat to pretend it is bacon—she calls it poor man's turkey. I know a man who holds a very minor political job because "he speeched around all over the country before election." I know another whose sole gardening effort is to scrape off the sod on a place about three feet square. On the resulting hard yellow clay, he arranged white-washed bricks to form his own initials.

I know one who hangs out a sign Clutch Specialist in a village of twenty-five houses, and I doubt if he's ever heard of the overworked mouse trap. I know one who aspires to the Beautiful Things of Life who, when she saw my garden in winter, said rapturously, "I bet this smells just like a beauty parlor in the summer." (I have regal lilies on my desk as I write—they do not give me nostalgia for beauty parlors.)

And I know a little girl who lives with a family of eleven others in a small shack with one bedroom, and she told me with a smile as glowing as the beam of sunlight that breaks through the storm cloud, "It's a tight fit but we sure get along fine."

No, Jerry is not a Specialist, but a woman patient nearly divorced her husband because he had Jerry for his own personal 'doctorin'' yet made her go to another M.D. so she knew he wanted her to die. Another young woman begged him to be present during her operation so that everything possible would be allowed to remain, as was, in her interior. When questioned, she implored, "Don't let them remove my O-VAR-ies, Doctor. I don't want to be a missionary to the heathen."

I saw him bathe a two-months-old dirt-encrusted rickety little baby who had never had a bath because it was winter. He spent a night with a kind elderly man during a heart attack. The next day the man said wearily, "You kept me alive last night and I appreciate it, Doctor, but the next time, let me rest. You do not know how welcome Death can be. It will be the finest experience of my life."

Jerry knows one who found and married a handsomer man, yet she returns regularly to bathe the previous husband and care for his house.
"Not a Specialist, but he can often diagnose disorders in various sections of the anatomy, bad tonsils, pregnancies, rampaging gall bladders, fractures, misplaced miscellaneous, flat feet, without calling in a separate consultant for each one—though happily, he can recognize his own limitations. The variety of situations and types of illnesses tax all his ingenuity, diagnostic skill, and endurance.

He has a case that was the victim of frequent D.T.'s. After the last spell, Jerry talked to him for hours, told him that his son was so ashamed of his father that he was becoming neurotic, wouldn't play with other boys, and was ashamed to bring them home. Jerry urged him to send his wife and son away and then go to the devil as soon as he could without humiliating them. Two weeks later the wife called by phone. "What did you say to Frank? He's been sober ever since. It is my first relief in eight years. Last night Johnny brought two boys home to supper. I feel like a new woman."

Jerry loves it. Why be a Specialist?

A sense of humor is blessed equipment for country medical practice. Not long ago, Jerry developed a complex about a new suit. He finally decided he could spare the time and cash and asked me to go with him to help select it. En route, the car broke down and cost the price of a new suit. We returned home slightly frayed as to nerves and cuffs but laughing and solvent.

Once a patient came, dead drunk, and paid a bill of ancient vintage, which deed we heard through the village grapevine, he regretted in his first sober moment. Only with difficulty was he persuaded that he had gone to such dire lengths during an unguarded moment in his cups.

They tell us that at the time of the draft, a local man was taken to register by his fond mama who told the board, "You dassan't take him. He has a fallen womb, flat arches, false teeth, hookworm, and two bad ovaries." He had a long service overseas and spent all his bonus within a week after he had received it.

I wouldn't have missed the time when Howard, at sixteen, was visibly affected by a heartrending scene in a movie sequence and said disgustedly as we came out, "And I thought my emotional days were over." Or his favorite expression, "Let the mountain come to Jehovah."

I like to remember, but could have missed the experience gladly, the time our dog, in super-playful mood, with eight healthy, appetizing children to select from, chose to bite the daughter of one of the few non-friendly families in town.

I am glad that I admitted a patient to speak to Jerry at the time when I had arrived at the rash and desperate conclusion that we must have new rugs and curtains. Life could not go on without them. While he waited to see Jerry, his eyes roved over the modest room and finally, he spoke in a hushed voice, "Excuse me, Miss, but you won't have to die to get to Heaven, will you?" I did not buy the rugs or curtains.

The phone, of necessity, sits by Jerry's elbow while we eat. The conversations do not always stimulate the appetite. When Nancy was not yet six, we once had very special company, and the phone, as usual, rang stridently. Nancy sighed and meekly volunteered, "Oh, dear, urine for lunch and bowels for dinner." Which is too literal to be very funny.

Nine out of ten of our plans go awry or just don't go at all. Many meals are delayed or never eaten. A large percentage of our work is necessarily for charity, so much so that I am apt to see amounts people owe, emblazoned on them like the Scarlet Letter, and only great self-control keeps me from greeting them, "How Do you Do, Mrs. $14.50?" Or, "Isn't this perfect weather, Mr. $39.00—a liberal discount for cash."

Cornelia Cattell Thompson

A Sonnet

I would not be absolved of humble tasks—
the watering of a small plant that holds in its
young tendrils a promise of green summer;
the winding of the tall clock that voices approval
as it stands guard over our household gods;
the dusting of fine old furniture whose sheen has
come through faithful service;
the pouring of tea from an old Spode pot that speaks
eloquently of the beauty of age;
the stirring of a fire that breathes life into our
little room with its varying shadows;
the lighting of lamps when evening, with quiet darkness,
surrounds us with gentle and protecting arms;
the bathing of a little child whose eyes make one forget
that older children can lack faith in one another;
These I would cherish and hold steady while the world rocks
on its axis.

We constantly face the realities of closed minds, great loyalties, poverty, birth, heroism, death, murder, incest, love, ignorance—but the most trying of these are closed minds and ignorance, We have little time or wherewithal to travel. But, like the mother of the fourteen fatherless children, we have put our minds to it and find infinitely satisfactory compensations.

I tell you truly, I wouldn't change it if I could.

—Appendix—

Cornelia Cattell Thompson Chronology

On February 5th, 1898, Cornelia Cattell Thompson was **born** in Wheeling, West Virginia, and soon moved to Martins Ferry, Ohio in **1900**, then on to Mount Pleasant, Ohio in **1906** where she was educated.

Cornelia's father, William Mahlon Cattell **(July 25, 1860-April 16, 1931)** came from a long line of Quakers, yet in 1893 he asked to be released from his Quaker church in Mount Pleasant. He wished to marry Edith Virginia Brenneman, a non-Quaker, and marrying outside the faith was grounds for disownment. For a time, they lived in Wheeling, West Virginia, where Cornelia and her brother Ezra were born. They moved to Martins Ferry, Ohio, in 1900. In **1906** William, a banker, moved his family back to Mount Pleasant where he and his family rejoined the Quaker faith.

In 1913 Cornelia's mother, Edith, died of cancer. A short time later, William once again moved his family, this time to nearby Smithfield, Ohio. Cornelia's oldest brother, Ezra, whom she adored, died during **WWI** in France where he is buried. Third in succession was brother Richard, who was a world-renowned surgeon. Next, was William Maurice, who moved to Portland, Oregon. William also served during **WWI**. Sister Edith died in **1905** at age 2. The youngest, Charles, would move to Chicago where he worked for Goodyear Tire and Rubber.

In **1917** Cornelia graduated at the head of her class from Mount Union College in Alliance, Ohio. After graduation, she taught school, first in Carrollton, Ohio, and last in Barnesville, Ohio.

While living in Smithfield, she met Dr. Jay Ira Thompson whom she would marry on **September 17, 1924.** Dr. Jay Thompson was born on **March 27th, 1890** near Steubenville, Ohio where his father worked in the steel mill. In **1914** he graduated from Ohio Medical School at Ohio University. He was married once before his marriage to Cornelia. Both his first wife, Doris Bailie and their child, died a few days apart in November **1919** (child stillborn, mother possibly from Spanish flu).

After her marriage to Doctor Jerry, Cornelia stopped teaching school though she continued teaching piano to children in Smithfield and presenting their recitals. She wrote most of her life, including children's books, articles, and this unpublished memoir which she donated to the Historical Society of Mount Pleasant. She also opened a collectable antique and craft shop in an adjacent property to their home on Maple Ave., Smithfield.

Jan. 31st, 1928, Jerry and Cornelia's daughter, Nancy Cornelia Thompson, was **born.**

Born **July 12th, 1918,** Howard Richard Fisher, following his parents' deaths, became the ward of Cornelia and Jerry Thompson. He graduated fom Smithfield High School, attended college and served in the US Navy during **WWII.** After the war, he was an accountant for the US government. Howard died of a heart attack in **1984**, at the age of 66. He donated his body to the UNC School of Medicine in Chapel Hill, North Carolina, near his home in Pinehurst.

On Oct. 17, 1955, Jerry, as Cornelia called him, after a long career as a country doctor, passed away. Daughter Nancy would die on **Oct. 24th, 1983,** just a year after her mother Cornelia's death.

On **June 1st, 1982** Cornelia passed away in Steubenville, Ohio, at the age of 84 and was buried alongside husband Jerry and other family at Mount Pleasant's Short Creek Cemetery.

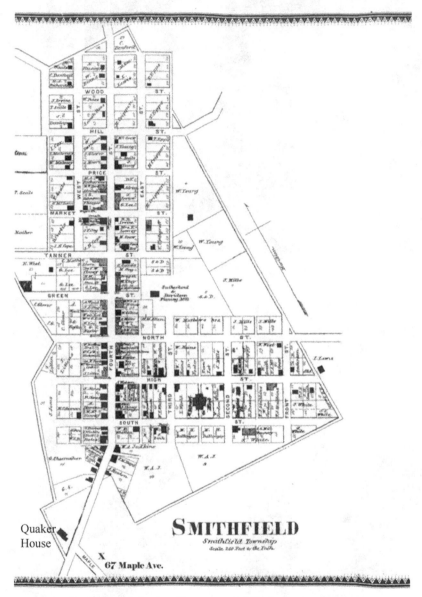

Quaker
House

SMITHFIELD

Smithfield Township
Scale. 240 Feet to the Inch

X
67 Maple Ave.

Smithfield Meeting House and 67 Maple Ave. home
lower left

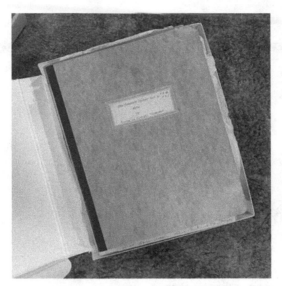

Whole manuscript and sample page

Typed manuscript page

Our greatest tragedy is the wanton destruction by the so-called strip mines. Acre after acre has been gutted, the land permanently ruined. The dirt is stripped off so that the coal can be scooped up with shovels. Everything in the path of the coal vein is destroyed. Great oak woods have been felled. I cannot express what a shock it is to return to a favorite woods and find it gone, as we have done several times. Farms are ruined. Farmhouse after farmhouse stands vacant because the land is no longer tillable. The land is valueless when they have removed the coal and left mile after mile of serpentine gaping wounds. The latest news is that one of the companies is bringing in a shovel that will move over 300 bushels at one gulp. (It is here.) I have not seen lands desolated by modern warfare but it would require a tremendous amount of bombs to wreak the desolation of just one of the "sunshine mines". I shudder to think that the Divine Plan which so obviously produced Ohio with its lovely hills, valleys, woods and streams, can be so ruthlessly defied.

We have the poor with us. We have the W.P.A. in generous numbers. We also have the W.O.O. (without obvious occupation - past or present). Many of these have never been known to work. They drape themselves at various intersections near the center of the village and busy themselves with nothing more constructive than a process of gradually changing the color of the cement. How they keep so plentifully supplied with tobacco is a mystery.

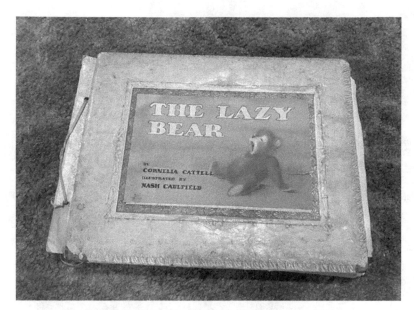

Children's book The Lazy Bear and handwritten
"Spring" Poem

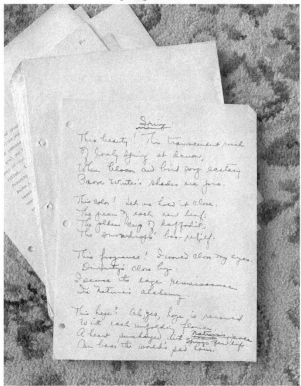

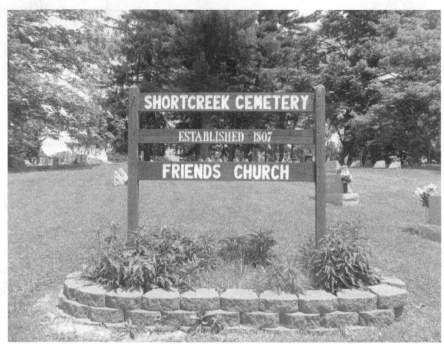

Grave sites of Thompson and Cattelle family in
Mount Pleasant, Ohio

Angela Feenerty is a research historian who was born in south-central Kentucky where her family instilled in her the love of history and gardening. She and her husband live on a farm in Martins Ferry, Ohio, where they raise and promote heritage livestock breeds. Together they founded the Heritage Dance Association, a group dedicated to preserving historic dance and music. Angela is President of the Historical Society of Mt Pleasant Ohio, a historic community with deep roots in the Quaker history. She has presented programs to various groups about Mt. Pleasant's historic past, highlighting the Underground Railroad and abolition of slavery. She has been published in *The Upper Ohio Valley Historical Review* on "Emancipated and Escaped Slaves and Freedmen of Mt. Pleasant, Ohio," and manages Ohio History Connection's Ohio Yearly Meeting House.

Larry Smith is a professor emeritus of Firelands College of Bowling Green State University where he taught literature and writing. He is also the director of Bottom Dog Press/ Bird Dog Publishing, a nonprofit literary organization in its 35th year. He is the author of poetry, fiction, memoir, and two literary biographies and films. He grew up 15 miles east of this book's setting of Smithfield in the steel mill town of Mingo Junction, Ohio.

Bottom Dog Press
Appalachian Writing Series

Appalachian Writing Series Anthologies

Free Shipping.
http://smithdocs.net

BIRD DOG PUBLISHING

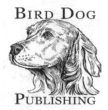

BIRD DOG

PUBLISHING

Lost and Found in Alaska: Memoir by Joel Rudinger 240 pgs. $18
Mingo Town & Memories by Larry Smith 96 pgs. $15
Trophy Kill by R. J. Norgard 256 pgs. $16
Symphonia Judaica: Jewish Symphony and Other Poems
by Joel Rudinger 117 pgs. $16
Words Walk: Poems by Ronald M. Ruble 168 pgs. $16
Homegoing by Michael Olin-Hitt 180 pgs. $16
A Wonderful Stupid Man: Stories by Allen Frost 190 pgs. $16
A Poetic Journey, Poems by Robert A. Reynolds, 86 pgs. $16
Dogs and Other Poems by Paul Piper, 80 pgs. $15
The Mermaid Translation by Allen Frost, 140 pgs. $15
Heart Murmurs: Poems by John Vanek, 120 pgs. $15
Home Recordings: Tales and Poems by Allen Frost. $14
A Life in Poems by William C. Wright, $10
Faces and Voices: Tales by Larry Smith, 136 pgs. $14
Second Story Woman: A Memoir of Second Chances
by Carole Calladine, 226 pgs. $15
256 Zones of Gray: Poems by Rob Smith, 80 pgs. $14
Another Life: Collected Poems by Allen Frost, 176 pgs. $14
Winter Apples: Poems by Paul S. Piper, 88 pgs. $14
Lake Effect: Poems by Laura Treacy Bentley, 108 pgs. $14
Depression Days on an Appalachian Farm: Poems
by Robert L. Tener, 80 pgs. $14
120 Charles Street, The Village: Journals & Other Writings 1949-1950
by Holly Beye, 240 pgs. $15

BIRD DOG PUBLISHING
A division of Bottom Dog Press, Inc.
Order Online at:
http://smithdocs.net/BirdDogy/BirdDogPage.html